The Complete Gastroparesis Diet Cookbook

1600 Days of Delicious, Nourishing, & Easy-to-Prepare Recipes to Reverse Gastroparesis, Acid Reflux, and Nausea. Includes a 30-Day Meal Plan

Kathleen H. Jensen

CONTENTS

Introduction 1

Chapter 1 3

Causes of Gastroparesis 3

Symptoms of Gastroparesis 3

Diagnosing Gastroparesis 4

Gastroparesis and Its Impact on Dietary Choices 4

Chapter 2 5

Managing Symptoms 5

Digestibility 5

Managing blood sugar levels... 5

Preventing Malnutrition 6

Meal Planning and Adaptation 6

Chapter 3 7

BREAKFAST 9

Pumpkin Spice Smoothie... 9

Baked Quinoa Breakfast Bars 10

Coconut Rice Pudding.. 12

Scrambled Eggs with Fresh Dill 13

Chia Seed and Raspberry Parfait 14

Creamy Polenta with Berries... 15

Poached Chicken and Rice Soup... 17

Spinach and Feta Omelette 18

Creamy Peanut Butter Porridge 19

Cinnamon Raisin French Toast (Gluten-Free)............................... 21

Creamy Oatmeal with Mashed Banana 22

Scrambled Tofu with Spinach.. 23

Baked Apples with Cinnamon 24

Quinoa Porridge with Almond Butter 26

Ginger Carrot Smoothie 27

Poached Egg with Steamed Asparagus 28

Blueberry Chia Pudding 30

Sweet Potato Hash Browns 31

SOUPS 34

Creamy Spinach and Potato Soup 34

Cilantro Lime Chicken Soup 35

Roasted Red Pepper and Tomato Bisque 36

Shrimp and Quinoa Chowder 38

Creamy Parsnip and Apple Soup 39

Lemon Chicken and Rice Soup 41

White Bean and Kale Soup 42

Creamy Mushroom and Rice Soup 44

Sweet Potato and Leek Soup 45

Turkey Meatball Soup with Rice 46

Butternut Squash Soup with Ginger 48

Chicken and Rice Congee 50

Creamy Tomato Soup with Rice 52

Miso Soup with Silken Tofu 53

Potato Leek Soup with a Hint of Nutmeg 54

Lentil and Spinach Stew 56

Turkey and Vegetable Broth 57

Creamy Cauliflower Soup 58

SALADS 61

Spinach and Quinoa Salad with Lemon Dressing 61

Shredded Carrot and Apple Salad 62

Tofu and Broccoli Slaw Salad 64

Pear and Walnut Salad 65

Roasted Beet and Arugula Salad 67

Grape and Cottage Cheese Salad 68

Caprese Salad with Balsamic Glaze 70

Jicama and Cucumber Salad 71

Thai-Inspired Cabbage Salad 72

Mixed Greens with Raspberry Walnut Vinaigrette 74

Mixed Greens with Grilled Chicken and Raspberry Vinaigrette 75

Avocado and Grapefruit Salad 77

Quinoa and Roasted Vegetable Salad 79

Cucumber and Mint Salad 80

Tuna Salad with Greek Yogurt Dressing 82

Beet and Orange Salad 84

Spinach and Strawberry Salad 85

Watermelon and Feta Salad 87

MAIN COURSES 89

Lemon Dill Baked Cod 89

Turkey and Quinoa Stuffed Bell Peppers 90

Creamy Chicken and Rice Casserole 92

Zucchini and Carrot Noodles with Pesto 94

Ginger Teriyaki Tofu 95

Baked Eggplant Parmesan (Gluten-Free) 97

Spinach and Feta Stuffed Chicken Breast 98

Lentil and Butternut Squash Curry 100

Baked Trout with Herbed Butter 102

Shrimp Scampi with Zoodles 103

Baked Salmon with Lemon-Dill Sauce 105

Turkey and Rice Casserole 106

Zucchini Noodles with Pesto 108

Baked Cod with Herbed Butter 109

Quiche with a Gluten-Free Crust...110

SIDE DISHES 113

Mashed Sweet Potatoes with Cinnamon 113

Roasted Brussels Sprouts with Pecans 114

Sautéed Green Beans with Almonds 115

Lemon Herb Quinoa Salad 116

Lemon Herb Quinoa Salad 118

Grilled Asparagus with Garlic Butter 119

Steamed Artichokes with Lemon Aioli...............................120

Mashed Turnips with Chives 122

Creamy Corn Pudding 123

Garlic Mashed Potatoes 124

Steamed Broccoli with Almonds 126

Sautéed Spinach with Garlic 127

Roasted Carrots with Dill 128

Mashed Cauliflower with Chives 130

Ginger Glazed Carrots 131

Lemon Herb Quinoa 132

Sliced Cucumber with Yogurt Dill Sauce 134

SNACKS..136

Baked Cinnamon Apple Slices 136

Rice Cakes with Cottage Cheese and Berries.....................137

Roasted Pumpkin Seeds with Sea Salt................................138

Peach and Banana Smoothie..139

Greek Yogurt Parfait with Kiwi...140

Almond Flour Banana Muffins 141

Cucumber and Bell Pepper Sticks with Hummus...............142

Baked Sweet Potato Fries 143

Cheddar Cheese Slices with Sliced Pear.............................144

Watermelon and Mint Skewers 145

Rice Cakes with Almond Butter 146

Banana and Peanut Butter Smoothie 147

Roasted Chickpeas with Paprika 148

Cottage Cheese with Pineapple 149

Greek Yogurt with Honey and Berries 150

Baked Apple Chips... 151

Carrot and Celery Sticks with Hummus 153

Boiled Edamame with Sea Salt..154

DESSERTS 156

Almond Flour Chocolate Chip Cookies 156

Chia Seed and Coconut Pudding 157

Baked Cinnamon Pears 158

Chocolate Avocado Brownies (Gluten-Free)...............................160

Coconut Rice Pudding with Mango 161

Lemon Sorbet 163

Vanilla Almond Milkshake 164

Raspberry and Dark Chocolate Yogurt Cups............................. 165

Blueberry Crumble (Gluten-Free) 166

Banana and Coconut Ice Cream.. 168

Rice Pudding with Cinnamon 169

Banana Ice Cream... 170

Chia Seed Pudding with Mango..172

Baked Pear with Caramel Drizzle...173

Almond Flour Blueberry Muffins 175

Coconut Milk Rice Pudding..176

Chocolate Avocado Mousse 177

Pumpkin Pie with a Gluten-Free Crust 179

BEVERAGES 181

Minty Cucumber and Melon Cooler 181

Raspberry Lemonade.. 182

Spinach and Pineapple Smoothie.. 183

Blueberry and Lavender Infused Water 185

Golden Milk Iced Latte 186

Cranberry and Orange Mocktail..187

Fresh Ginger and Lemon Tea 189

Papaya and Mango Smoothie 190

Sparkling Lavender Lemonade 191

Green Tea Latte with Almond Milk.. 193

Lemon Water with Fresh Mint.. 194

Cucumber and Mint Infused Water 195

Berry Smoothie with Spinach...196

Iced Green Tea with Honey 198

Golden Milk (Turmeric Latte)..199

Fresh Orange and Carrot Juice 200

Cranberry and Raspberry Sparkling Water..............................201

Chapter 12 204

Week 1... 204

Week 2 205

Week 3 206

Week 4 207

Conclusion.. 209

Recipe Index 210

Introduction

Navigating Your Journey to Wellness

This cookbook serves as a guide for individuals living with gastroparesis, offering not only a collection of recipes but also tips and strategies to enhance their quality of life and manage the condition more effectively. If you or someone you care about is affected by this condition, you may be familiar with the challenges it can bring. Gastroparesis is a condition where the stomach takes longer than usual to empty its contents. It can lead to various symptoms, including nausea, vomiting, abdominal pain, and a sensation of fullness, even after eating a small amount of food.

Living with gastroparesis can present challenges, but it's important to remember that you can still enjoy meals that are both delicious and nutritious. This cookbook aims to assist you in managing a gastroparesis diet by offering a range of thoughtfully created recipes that are easy on your digestive system and enjoyable to eat.

In these pages, you will find various recipes specifically developed for individuals with gastroparesis. Whether you've recently been diagnosed, have been living with this condition for some time, or are a caregiver looking to prepare suitable meals, this cookbook offers a variety of recipes that cater to different needs.

The process of developing these recipes started by gaining a thorough understanding of gastroparesis, including its symptoms and dietary needs. Managing your condition involves more than just avoiding specific foods; it also involves finding enjoyment in the foods you can eat. The recipes provided are designed to help you enjoy meals without worsening your symptoms. You'll find a variety of dishes that are easy on the stomach while still being flavorful and nutritious.

The cookbook is organized into chapters that cover various aspects of a diet suitable for individuals with gastroparesis. We have covered a range of soft and comforting foods that can help soothe your stomach, as well as low-fiber options that are easier to digest. You can also find inspiration in liquid and pureed dishes and learn how to create small, frequent meals that are gentle on your digestive system. Our section on easy-to-digest desserts offers guilt-free indulgence for those who enjoy sweet treats.

This cookbook aims to provide you with a positive and empowering experience as you cook and enjoy meals from this cookbook. You're not alone on this journey, and hopefully, *"The Complete Gastroparesis Cookbook,"* will be a helpful resource for delicious gastroparesis-friendly recipes.

As you begin this culinary journey, we encourage you to explore the various possibilities and adjust the recipes according to your taste. While these recipes are designed to accommodate individuals with gastroparesis, we acknowledge that individual needs and preferences may differ. Feel free to make modifications to suit your specific needs and personalize these recipes.

Remember that this cookbook is not only a compilation of recipes but also a resource to assist you in improving your quality of life while managing gastroparesis. We aim to offer inspiration, delicious meals, and a sense of community to support your journey towards better digestive health. May you find joy in the process of creating and savoring these dishes, and may your journey towards wellness be filled with nourishment and self-care.

Let's embark on a culinary journey together, where every meal is an opportunity to nourish your body, delight your senses, and contribute to your overall well-being.

Chapter 1

Understanding Gastroparesis

Gastroparesis, also known as "paralyzed stomach," is a gastrointestinal disorder that impairs the normal movement and emptying of food from the stomach into the small intestine. It is a condition that can have a significant impact on one's quality of life, causing a variety of uncomfortable and occasionally debilitating symptoms. In this section, we'll discuss the fundamental aspects of gastroparesis, including its causes, symptoms, diagnosis, and impact on dietary choices.

Causes of Gastroparesis

Gastroparesis can have multiple underlying causes. Damage to the vagus nerve is a potential cause, as it plays a vital role in regulating stomach muscles. Damage can occur due to various factors, including diabetes, surgical procedures involving the stomach or vagus nerve, viral infections, or certain medications. Idiopathic gastroparesis is a condition where the exact cause is unknown and can develop in specific individuals. Gastroparesis is characterized by impaired stomach muscle function, which can result in slowed or disrupted digestion. The cause of gastroparesis can vary.

Symptoms of Gastroparesis

Gastroparesis can trigger a range of symptoms, which can vary in severity. Common symptoms include:

1. **Nausea:** The persistent or recurrent sensation of queasiness.
2. **Vomiting:** It can be distressing and unpredictable.
3. **Abdominal Discomfort:** A feeling of fullness or bloating that persists even after eating small amounts of food.
4. **Heartburn:** Stomach acid can flow back into the esophagus due to delayed stomach emptying, causing discomfort.
5. **Erratic Blood Sugar Levels:** Particularly among individuals with diabetes, erratic blood sugar levels can occur due to gastroparesis.
    1. These symptoms have the potential to significantly disrupt daily life, making it challenging to enjoy regular meals or social occasions that revolve around food.

Diagnosing Gastroparesis

If you experience any of the symptoms mentioned earlier, it is vital to seek advice from a healthcare professional. Diagnosing gastroparesis usually requires a combination of medical history, physical examination, and specific tests. A gastric emptying study is a standard diagnostic tool for gastroparesis, and it is used to track the rate at which the stomach empties. It involves consuming a meal that contains a small amount of a radioactive substance, which enables medical professionals to monitor the process accurately.

Gastroparesis and Its Impact on Dietary Choices

Gastroparesis significantly affects what and how you are able to eat. Dietary choices are essential for managing the condition because the stomach's ability to process food is compromised. A gastroparesis-friendly diet emphasizes foods that are easier to digest, including low-fiber options, and encourages smaller, more frequent meals. Liquid and pureed foods can be beneficial.

When dealing with gastroparesis, it's important to remember that everyone's experience with the condition is unique as you explore the culinary landscape. What works for one individual may not work for another. This cookbook offers a variety of recipes specifically designed for individuals with gastroparesis. It aims to help you discover and enjoy dishes that align with your preferences and dietary needs.

Understanding gastroparesis is a critical step in effectively managing the condition. By educating yourself about the condition and understanding its impact on your body, you can make informed choices, such as dietary decisions, to enhance your overall well-being. This cookbook aims to provide a valuable resource for individuals seeking better health by offering a wide range of delicious recipes that cater to the specific dietary requirements of individuals with gastroparesis. We hope that this knowledge empowers you to take control of your health and enjoy meals that are both nourishing and enjoyable.

Chapter 2

The Significance of Diet in Managing Gastroparesis

The role of diet in managing gastroparesis is significant. The diet and eating habits of individuals with this condition can have a considerable impact on their quality of life. Gastroparesis is a condition characterized by delayed stomach emptying. It can present unique challenges, but following a carefully crafted diet can help alleviate symptoms, improve comfort, and promote overall well-being. In this section, we will explore the critical role that diet plays in managing gastroparesis effectively.

Managing Symptoms

The main objective of a gastroparesis-specific diet is to manage and relieve the unpleasant symptoms linked to the condition. Nausea, vomiting, bloating, and abdominal discomfort are common issues that can significantly affect daily life. Making appropriate dietary choices effectively decreases the frequency and severity of these symptoms.

Digestibility

Digestibility refers to the ability of a substance to be broken down and absorbed by the body. Gastroparesis is a condition that affects the stomach's ability to break down and process food efficiently. Certain foods, especially those that are high in fiber or fat, can worsen symptoms. A gastroparesis-friendly diet includes foods that are easy to digest, such as well-cooked vegetables, lean proteins, and low-fiber grains. These choices can potentially help prevent food from remaining in the stomach for a long time, which may reduce discomfort and the likelihood of complications.

Managing blood sugar levels

Managing blood sugar levels is an essential aspect of gastroparesis care for individuals with diabetes. Erratic blood sugar fluctuations can occur due to unpredictable digestion in this condition. A personalized diet can assist in stabilizing blood sugar levels by focusing on eating small, frequent meals and managing carbohydrate intake.

Preventing Malnutrition

Gastroparesis may hinder the absorption of essential nutrients from food, potentially leading to malnutrition. A well-balanced diet can provide the necessary nutrients and energy to prevent deficiencies and support the healing process. Healthcare professionals may recommend supplements in certain situations to help ensure that the body receives essential vitamins and minerals.

Meal Planning and Adaptation

The management of gastroparesis varies depending on the individual and does not follow a universal approach. Individuals may have different tolerances for specific foods, and the severity of symptoms can vary. A diet customized to your specific needs and sensitivities is essential. This cookbook is designed to be flexible, allowing you to modify recipes according to your preferences and current circumstances. Working with healthcare professionals and keeping a food diary can help identify trigger foods and create a personalized meal plan.

In summary, the importance of diet in managing gastroparesis cannot be overstated. A well-balanced diet can help manage symptoms, promote overall health, and improve your quality of life. By making informed food choices and working closely with your healthcare team, you can effectively manage gastroparesis and enjoy delicious, nourishing meals that are less likely to worsen your condition. This cookbook serves as a guide to help you make choices suitable for gastroparesis, providing a variety of recipes that are friendly to your digestive health. It aims to make your journey towards better digestive health enjoyable and fulfilling.

Chapter 3

Understanding the Gastroparesis Diet

Starting a gastroparesis diet may seem overwhelming, but it can lead to better health and help manage symptoms. Successfully following this diet involves:

- Gaining knowledge about your body.
- Consciously selecting food options.
- Developing a different approach to your relationship with food.

Here, we'll discuss some essential strategies for effectively managing the gastroparesis diet.

1. **Educate Yourself:** The first step is to become well-informed about gastroparesis and its dietary implications. Understanding the condition and its impact on your digestive system will enable you to make well-informed decisions about your diet.
2. **Work with Healthcare Professionals:** Work together with a healthcare team that specializes in gastroenterology or nutrition to work together. They can assist you in developing a customized gastroparesis diet plan tailored to your specific needs and preferences.
3. **Keep a Food Diary:** Tracking your meals and symptoms can be very helpful. A food diary can help identify trigger foods that may worsen your symptoms and guide you in making appropriate adjustments to your diet.
4. **Commence Slowly:** When transitioning to a diet suitable for gastroparesis, it is advisable to introduce changes gradually. Start with smaller, more frequent meals and opt for softer, easily digestible foods. The gradual shift can make the adjustment easier for your body.
5. **Experiment with Recipes:** Explore the recipes in this cookbook and modify them according to your preferences. Having gastroparesis doesn't necessarily mean you have to compromise on flavor. By employing creativity and flexibility, it is possible to savor delectable and nutritious meals.

6. **Portion Control:** Maintain moderate portions to avoid overloading your stomach. Consuming smaller meals can alleviate strain on your digestive system and decrease discomfort.
7. **Stay Hydrated:** Remember to drink water regularly throughout the day to prevent dehydration. Proper hydration is vital for digestion and overall health.
8. **Listen to Your Body:** Be mindful of how your body reacts to various foods. If a specific meal causes discomfort, make changes to your diet accordingly. Your body's signals can be a helpful guide.

Successfully following the gastroparesis diet requires patience and adaptability. It's a process of self-discovery and empowerment. By making thoughtful choices, seeking professional guidance, and trying out new recipes, you can effectively manage your condition and find joy in nourishing your body while reducing symptoms. This cookbook aims to assist you throughout your cooking journey by offering a variety of recipes that are suitable for individuals with gastroparesis. These recipes are designed to make your culinary experience enjoyable and satisfying.

BREAKFAST

Pumpkin Spice Smoothie

Prep Time: 5 minutes
Cook Time: 0 minutes
Number of Servings: 2

Ingredients:

- 1 cup canned pumpkin puree
- 1 ripe banana, peeled and sliced
- 1/2 cup plain Greek yogurt
- 1/2 cup unsweetened almond milk
- 1/4 cup old-fashioned rolled oats
- 1 tablespoon honey
- 1/2 teaspoon ground cinnamon
- 1/4 teaspoon ground nutmeg
- 1/4 teaspoon ground ginger
- 1/4 teaspoon ground cloves
- 1/4 teaspoon vanilla extract
- Ice cubes (optional)

Instructions:

1. In a blender, add one cup of canned pumpkin puree, 1 sliced ripe banana, 1/2 cup of plain Greek yogurt, 1/2 cup of unsweetened almond milk, 1/4 cup of old-fashioned rolled oats, one tablespoon of honey, 1/2 teaspoon of ground cinnamon, 1/4 teaspoon of ground nutmeg, 1/4 teaspoon of ground ginger, 1/4 teaspoon of ground cloves, and 1/4 teaspoon of vanilla extract.

2. If desired, add a few ice cubes for a colder smoothie.

3. Blend all the ingredients until smooth and well combined.

4. Pour the pumpkin spice smoothie into glasses and serve immediately.

Nutritional Information (per serving):

- Carbs: 33 grams

- Fats: 4 grams

- Fiber: 5 grams

- Sodium: 78 milligrams

- Protein: 6 grams

Baked Quinoa Breakfast Bars

Prep Time: 15 minutes
Cook Time: 35 minutes
Number of Servings: 12 bars

Ingredients:

- 1 cup quinoa, rinsed and drained

- 2 cups unsweetened almond milk

- 1/4 cup honey

- 2 large eggs

- 1 teaspoon vanilla extract

- 1/2 teaspoon ground cinnamon

- 1/4 teaspoon salt

- 1/2 cup dried cranberries

- 1/4 cup chopped walnuts

- 1/4 cup shredded unsweetened coconut

- 1/4 cup mini chocolate chips (optional)

Instructions:

1. Turn on your oven and set it to 350°F (175°C) and grease an 8x8-inch (20x20 cm) baking dish.

2. In a saucepan, add one cup of rinsed and drained quinoa and two cups of unsweetened almond milk. Bring to a boil over medium heat. Once it boils, reduce the heat to low, cover, and simmer for 15-20 minutes, or until the quinoa is cooked and the liquid is absorbed. Take it out from heat and let it cool slightly.

3. In a mixing bowl, whisk 1/4 cup of honey, 2 large eggs, one teaspoon of vanilla extract, 1/2 teaspoon of ground cinnamon, and 1/4 teaspoon of salt.

4. Add the cooked quinoa to the wet mixture and stir to combine.

5. Gently fold in 1/2 cup of dried cranberries, 1/4 cup of chopped walnuts, 1/4 cup of shredded unsweetened coconut, and 1/4 cup of mini chocolate chips (if using).

6. Pour the quinoa mixture into the greased baking dish, spreading it out evenly.

7. Bake in the preheated oven for 30-35 minutes, or until the edges are golden brown and the bars are set in the middle.

8. Remove from the oven and let the bars cool in the dish for about 10 minutes.

9. Using a sharp knife, cut the baked quinoa mixture into 12 bars.

10. Allow the bars to cool completely in the dish before removing and serving.

Nutritional Information (per bar):

- Carbs: 26 grams

- Fats: 6 grams

- Fiber: 3 grams

- Sodium: 102 milligrams

- Protein: 5 grams

Coconut Rice Pudding

Prep Time: 5 minutes
Cook Time: 40 minutes
Number of Servings: 4

Ingredients:

- 1 cup white rice

- 2 cups coconut milk (unsweetened)

- 1/4 cup honey

- 1/2 teaspoon vanilla extract

- 1/4 teaspoon salt

- 1/4 cup shredded coconut (unsweetened)

- 1/4 cup chopped pineapple (canned in juice, drained)

- 1/4 cup sliced almonds

Instructions:

1. In a medium-sized saucepan, add one cup of white rice and two cups of unsweetened coconut milk.

2. Bring the mixture to a boil over medium-high heat, then reduce the heat to low, cover, and simmer for about 20-25 minutes, or until the rice is tender and has absorbed most of the liquid.

3. Stir in 1/4 cup of honey, 1/2 teaspoon of vanilla extract, and 1/4 teaspoon of salt into the cooked rice. Keep on cooking over low heat for an extra 10 minutes, stirring occasionally, until the mixture thickens.

4. Take out the saucepan from heat and let the rice pudding cool slightly.

5. While the pudding is cooling, toast 1/4 cup of shredded unsweetened coconut in a dry skillet over medium heat until it turns golden brown, stirring frequently to prevent burning.

6. Once the rice pudding has cooled a bit, gently fold in the toasted coconut.

7. Divide the rice pudding into serving bowls and top each bowl with 1/4 cup of drained, chopped canned pineapple and 1/4 cup of sliced almonds.

8. Serve the coconut rice pudding warm or chilled.

Nutritional Information (per serving):

- Carbs: 59 grams

- Fats: 29 grams

- Fiber: 2 grams

- Sodium: 150 milligrams

- Protein: 7 grams

Scrambled Eggs with Fresh Dill

Prep Time: 5 minutes
Cook Time: 5 minutes
Number of Servings: 2

Ingredients:

- 4 large eggs

- 2 tablespoons unsalted butter

- 2 tablespoons fresh dill, finely chopped

- Salt and pepper, to taste

Instructions:

1. Crack 4 large eggs into a bowl and beat them well.

2. Heat a non-stick skillet over low to medium heat and add two tablespoons of unsalted butter. Allow the butter to melt and coat the bottom of the skillet evenly.

3. Pour the beaten eggs into the skillet and let them cook undisturbed for a few moments until they start to set around the edges.

4. Gently stir the eggs with a spatula, pushing them from the edges towards the center. Continue to stir and fold the eggs until mostly cooked but still slightly runny.

5. Sprinkle two tablespoons of finely chopped fresh dill evenly over the eggs. Keep on cooking and gently stir until the eggs are fully cooked and no longer runny.

6. Season the scrambled eggs with salt and pepper to taste.

7. Serve the scrambled eggs with fresh dill immediately.

Nutritional Information (per serving):

- Carbs: 0 grams

- Fats: 18 grams

- Fiber: 0 grams

- Sodium: 92 milligrams

- Protein: 12 grams

Chia Seed and Raspberry Parfait

Prep Time: 10 minutes
Cook Time: 0 minutes
Number of Servings: 2

Ingredients:

- 1/4 cup chia seeds

- 1 cup unsweetened almond milk

- 1 tablespoon honey

- 1/2 teaspoon vanilla extract

- 1 cup fresh raspberries

- 1/4 cup chopped almonds

Instructions:

1. In a mixing bowl, add 1/4 cup of chia seeds and one cup of unsweetened almond milk. Stir sufficiently to combine.

2. Add one tablespoon of honey and 1/2 teaspoon of vanilla extract to the chia seed mixture. Stir again to incorporate the sweetener and flavor.

3. Cover the bowl with plastic wrap or a lid and refrigerate for at least 2 hours, or overnight, to allow the chia seeds to absorb the liquid and create a pudding-like consistency.

4. Once the chia pudding has set, give it a good stir to ensure an even texture.

5. In serving glasses or bowls, layer the chia pudding with one cup of fresh raspberries and 1/4 cup of chopped almonds.

6. Repeat the layering process until the glasses are filled.

7. Finish with a few raspberries and a sprinkle of chopped almonds on top.

8. Serve the chia seed and raspberry parfait immediately or refrigerate until ready to eat.

Nutritional Information (per serving):

- Carbs: 30 grams

- Fats: 15 grams

- Fiber: 14 grams

- Sodium: 94 milligrams

- Protein: 8 grams

Creamy Polenta with Berries

Prep Time: 5 minutes
Cook Time: 30 minutes
Number of Servings: 4

Ingredients:

- 1 cup cornmeal (polenta)

- 4 cups water

- 1/4 cup honey

- 1/2 teaspoon vanilla extract
- 1/4 teaspoon salt
- 1 cup mixed berries (strawberries, blueberries, raspberries)
- 1/4 cup chopped almonds

Instructions:

1. In a medium-sized saucepan, bring 4 cups of water to a boil.
2. Gradually whisk in one cup of cornmeal (polenta) into the boiling water to avoid lumps.
3. Reduce the heat to low and simmer, stirring frequently, for approximately 25-30 minutes or until the polenta is thick and creamy. Add more water if needed to achieve the desired consistency.
4. Stir in 1/4 cup of honey, 1/2 teaspoon of vanilla extract, and 1/4 teaspoon of salt into the creamy polenta. Mix sufficiently.
5. Take out the polenta from the heat and let it cool slightly.
6. In serving bowls, spoon the creamy polenta evenly.
7. Top the polenta with one cup of mixed berries, including strawberries, blueberries, and raspberries.
8. Sprinkle 1/4 cup of chopped almonds over the berries.
9. Serve the creamy polenta with berries warm.

Nutritional Information (per serving):

- Carbs: 56 grams
- Fats: 11 grams
- Fiber: 6 grams
- Sodium: 150 milligrams
- Protein: 6 grams

Poached Chicken and Rice Soup

Prep Time: 10 minutes
Cook Time: 40 minutes
Number of Servings: 4

Ingredients:

- 1 pound boneless, skinless chicken breasts

- 1 cup white rice

- 6 cups low-sodium chicken broth

- 1 carrot, peeled and sliced

- 1 celery stalk, diced

- 1/2 cup green beans, trimmed and chopped

- 1/2 teaspoon dried thyme

- 1/2 teaspoon dried rosemary

- Salt and pepper, to taste

- Fresh parsley, for garnish

Instructions:

1. In a large pot, add 6 cups of low-sodium chicken broth, one cup of white rice, 1 peeled and sliced carrot, and 1 diced celery stalk.

2. Bring the mixture to a boil over medium-high heat.

3. Once boiling, add 1/2 teaspoon of dried thyme and 1/2 teaspoon of dried rosemary. Stir sufficiently.

4. Reduce the heat to low, cover the pot, and let it simmer for about 20 minutes, or until the rice is cooked and the vegetables are tender.

5. While the soup is simmering, poach 1 pound of boneless, skinless chicken breasts. To do this, place the chicken breasts in a separate saucepan and cover them with water. Bring the water to a boil, then reduce the heat to low, cover, and simmer for about 15-20 minutes, or until the chicken is properly cooked. Once cooked, take out the chicken from the water, let it cool slightly, and then shred it into bite-sized pieces.

6. Once the rice and vegetables in the soup are tender, add the shredded chicken and 1/2 cup of chopped green beans to the pot.

7. Season the soup with salt and pepper to taste. Adjust the seasoning as needed.

8. Continue to simmer the soup for an extra 5-10 minutes, or until the chicken and green beans are heated through.

9. Serve the poached chicken and rice soup hot, garnished with fresh parsley.

Nutritional Information (per serving):

- Carbs: 38 grams

- Fats: 3 grams

- Fiber: 2 grams

- Sodium: 490 milligrams

- Protein: 22 grams

Spinach and Feta Omelette

Prep Time: 5 minutes
Cook Time: 5 minutes
Number of Servings: 1

Ingredients:

- 2 large eggs

- 1/2 cup fresh spinach leaves, chopped

- 1/4 cup crumbled feta cheese

- 1/4 cup diced tomatoes

- 1/4 teaspoon dried oregano

- Salt and pepper, to taste

- 1 teaspoon olive oil

Instructions:

1. Crack 2 large eggs into a bowl and whisk them together until well beaten.

2. Heat one teaspoon of olive oil in a non-stick skillet over medium-low heat.

3. Add 1/2 cup of chopped fresh spinach leaves to the skillet. Cook for 1-2 minutes, or until the spinach wilts.

4. Pour the beaten eggs over the wilted spinach in the skillet.

5. Sprinkle 1/4 cup of crumbled feta cheese evenly over the eggs.

6. Add 1/4 cup of diced tomatoes on top of the cheese.

7. Sprinkle 1/4 teaspoon of dried oregano, salt, and pepper to taste over the ingredients in the skillet.

8. Cook the omelette for 2-3 minutes or until the edges are set.

9. Carefully fold the omelette in half with a spatula.

10. Keep on cooking for another 1-2 minutes, or until the omelette is properly cooked but still slightly moist on the inside.

11. Slide the spinach and feta omelette onto a plate and serve hot.

Nutritional Information (per serving):

- Carbs: 4 grams

- Fats: 16 grams

- Fiber: 1 gram

- Sodium: 433 milligrams

- Protein: 17 grams

Creamy Peanut Butter Porridge

Prep Time: 5 minutes
Cook Time: 10 minutes
Number of Servings: 2

Ingredients:

- 1 cup old-fashioned oats

- 2 cups water
- 2 tablespoons creamy peanut butter
- 1 tablespoon honey
- 1/4 teaspoon salt
- 1/4 cup chopped bananas
- 1/4 cup chopped strawberries

Instructions:

1. In a saucepan, add one cup of old-fashioned oats and two cups of water.

2. Bring the mixture to a boil over medium-high heat, stirring occasionally.

3. Reduce the heat to low and simmer for about 5-7 minutes, or until the oats are cooked and the porridge reaches your desired thickness.

4. Stir in two tablespoons of creamy peanut butter, one tablespoon of honey, and 1/4 teaspoon of salt into the cooked oats. Mix sufficiently until the peanut butter is fully incorporated.

5. Take out the porridge from heat and let it cool slightly.

6. In serving bowls, divide the creamy peanut butter porridge.

7. Top each bowl with 1/4 cup of chopped bananas and 1/4 cup of chopped strawberries.

8. Serve the peanut butter porridge warm.

Nutritional Information (per serving):

- Carbs: 46 grams
- Fats: 13 grams
- Fiber: 6 grams
- Sodium: 172 milligrams
- Protein: 9 grams

Cinnamon Raisin French Toast (Gluten-Free)

Prep Time: 10 minutes
Cook Time: 10 minutes
Number of Servings: 4

Ingredients:

- 8 slices gluten-free bread

- 2 large eggs

- 1/2 cup lactose-free milk

- 1 teaspoon ground cinnamon

- 1/4 teaspoon vanilla extract

- 1/4 cup raisins

- 1 tablespoon butter

- Maple syrup, for serving (optional)

Instructions:

1. In a shallow dish, whisk 2 large eggs, 1/2 cup of lactose-free milk, one teaspoon of ground cinnamon, and 1/4 teaspoon of vanilla extract.

2. Dip each of the 8 slices of gluten-free bread into the egg mixture, ensuring both sides are coated.

3. In a non-stick skillet, melt one tablespoon of butter over medium heat.

4. Place the dipped bread slices in the skillet and cook for about 2-3 minutes per side, or until golden brown and crispy.

5. While the French toast is cooking, sprinkle 1/4 cup of raisins evenly over the slices.

6. Once the French toast is cooked to your liking and the raisins are slightly plump, take them out from the skillet.

7. Serve the cinnamon raisin French toast warm, with maple syrup if desired.

Nutritional Information (per serving):

- Carbs: 31 grams

- Fats: 10 grams

- Fiber: 2 grams

- Sodium: 263 milligrams

- Protein: 7 grams

Creamy Oatmeal with Mashed Banana

Prep Time: 5 minutes
Cook Time: 10 minutes
Number of Servings: 2

Ingredients:

- 1 cup old-fashioned oats

- 2 cups water

- 2 ripe bananas, mashed

- 1/4 cup lactose-free milk

- 1/4 teaspoon ground cinnamon

- 1/4 teaspoon vanilla extract

- 1 tablespoon honey (optional)

- Sliced bananas and chopped walnuts for topping (optional)

Instructions:

1. In a saucepan, add one cup of old-fashioned oats and two cups of water.

2. Bring the mixture to a boil over medium-high heat, then reduce the heat to low and simmer for about 5-7 minutes, stirring occasionally, until the oats are tender and the mixture thickens.

3. While the oats are cooking, mash 2 ripe bananas in a bowl until smooth.

4. Once the oats are cooked, take out the saucepan from the heat.

5. Stir in the mashed bananas, 1/4 cup of lactose-free milk, 1/4 teaspoon of ground cinnamon, and 1/4 teaspoon of vanilla extract into the cooked oats. Mix sufficiently to combine all the ingredients.

6. If desired, add one tablespoon of honey for sweetness, adjusting to taste.

7. Serve the creamy oatmeal with mashed banana in bowls.

8. Top each serving with sliced bananas and chopped walnuts if you like.

Nutritional Information (per serving):

- Carbs: 54 grams

- Fats: 4 grams

- Fiber: 7 grams

- Sodium: 13 milligrams

- Protein: 6 grams

Scrambled Tofu with Spinach

Prep Time: 10 minutes
Cook Time: 15 minutes
Number of Servings: 2

Ingredients:

- 14 ounces firm tofu, crumbled

- 2 cups fresh spinach, chopped

- 1/2 onion, finely chopped

- 2 cloves garlic, minced

- 1/2 teaspoon ground turmeric

- 1/2 teaspoon ground cumin

- Salt and pepper, to taste

- 1 tablespoon olive oil

Instructions:

1. In a large skillet, heat one tablespoon of olive oil over medium heat.

2. Add 1/2 finely chopped onion and 2 cloves minced garlic to the skillet. Sauté for 2-3 minutes, or until the onion becomes translucent.

3. Add the crumbled tofu to the skillet. Sprinkle with 1/2 teaspoon of ground turmeric and 1/2 teaspoon of ground cumin. Season with salt and pepper to taste.

4. Cook the tofu mixture, stirring occasionally, for about 5-7 minutes, or until the tofu is heated through and begins to brown slightly.

5. Add two cups of chopped fresh spinach to the skillet. Keep on cooking, stirring, until the spinach wilts and blends with the tofu mixture. This should take about 2-3 minutes.

6. Taste and adjust the seasoning with more salt and pepper if needed.

7. Once the spinach is wilted and well combined with the tofu, take out the skillet from heat.

8. Serve the scrambled tofu with spinach hot, garnished with additional seasonings if desired.

Nutritional Information (per serving):

- Carbs: 7 grams

- Fats: 12 grams

- Fiber: 2 grams

- Sodium: 238 milligrams

- Protein: 11 grams

Baked Apples with Cinnamon

Prep Time: 10 minutes
Cook Time: 40 minutes
Number of Servings: 4

Ingredients:

- 4 medium-sized apples
- 2 tablespoons unsalted butter, melted
- 1/4 cup brown sugar
- 1 teaspoon ground cinnamon
- 1/4 teaspoon ground nutmeg
- 1/4 teaspoon ground cloves
- 1/4 cup chopped pecans (optional)
- 1/4 cup raisins (optional)
- 1/4 cup water

Instructions:

1. Turn on your oven and set it to 350°F (175°C).
2. Wash and core 4 medium-sized apples. Use a knife or an apple corer to take out the seeds and create a well in the center, leaving the bottom intact.
3. In a small bowl, mix together 1/4 cup of brown sugar, one teaspoon of ground cinnamon, 1/4 teaspoon of ground nutmeg, and 1/4 teaspoon of ground cloves.
4. In a separate bowl, melt two tablespoons of unsalted butter.
5. Brush the melted butter over the surface of each apple, using a pastry brush or a spoon.
6. Stuff each apple with the brown sugar and spice mixture, distributing it evenly among the apples.
7. If desired, fill each apple with 1/4 cup of chopped pecans and 1/4 cup of raisins.
8. Place the stuffed apples in a baking dish and add 1/4 cup of water to the bottom of the dish.
9. Cover the baking dish with aluminum foil.

10. Bake in the preheated oven for about 30-40 minutes, or until the apples are tender and can be easily pierced with a fork.

11. Serve the baked apples with cinnamon hot, with or without a scoop of vanilla ice cream or a dollop of whipped cream if desired.

Nutritional Information (per serving):

- Carbs: 42 grams

- Fats: 9 grams

- Fiber: 6 grams

- Sodium: 4 milligrams

- Protein: 1 gram

Quinoa Porridge with Almond Butter

Prep Time: 5 minutes
Cook Time: 15 minutes
Number of Servings: 2

Ingredients:

- 1/2 cup quinoa

- 1 1/2 cups lactose-free milk

- 2 tablespoons almond butter

- 1 tablespoon honey (optional)

- 1/2 teaspoon ground cinnamon

- 1/4 teaspoon vanilla extract

- Sliced almonds and banana slices for topping (optional)

Instructions:

1. Rinse 1/2 cup of quinoa under cold water until the water runs clear. This helps remove any bitter residue.

2. In a saucepan, add the rinsed quinoa and 1 1/2 cups of lactose-free milk.

3. Bring the mixture to a boil over medium-high heat.

4. Reduce the heat to low, cover the saucepan, and let it simmer for about 15 minutes, or until the quinoa is cooked and has absorbed most of the milk. Stir occasionally to prevent sticking.

5. Once the quinoa is cooked, take out the saucepan from heat.

6. Stir in two tablespoons of almond butter, one tablespoon of honey (if desired), 1/2 teaspoon of ground cinnamon, and 1/4 teaspoon of vanilla extract into the cooked quinoa. Mix sufficiently until all ingredients are fully incorporated.

7. Serve the quinoa porridge with almond butter hot.

8. If desired, top with sliced almonds and banana slices for added flavor and texture.

Nutritional Information (per serving):

- Carbs: 42 grams

- Fats: 12 grams

- Fiber: 5 grams

- Sodium: 82 milligrams

- Protein: 9 grams

Ginger Carrot Smoothie

Prep Time: 5 minutes
Cook Time: 0 minutes
Number of Servings: 2

Ingredients:

- 2 cups carrots, peeled and chopped

- 1 banana

- 1 cup lactose-free yogurt

- 1/2 teaspoon fresh ginger, grated

- 1 tablespoon honey (optional)

- 1/2 cup ice cubes

Instructions:

1. Peel and chop two cups of carrots.

2. In a blender, add the chopped carrots, 1 banana, one cup of lactose-free yogurt, 1/2 teaspoon of fresh grated ginger, and 1/2 cup of ice cubes.

3. If you prefer a sweeter taste, you can add one tablespoon of honey to the mixture.

4. Blend all the ingredients until the mixture is smooth and well combined. You may need to stop and scrape down the sides of the blender to ensure everything is blended evenly.

5. Once the ginger carrot smoothie is smooth and creamy, pour it into two serving glasses.

6. Serve the smoothie immediately for the best taste and texture.

Nutritional Information (per serving):

- Carbs: 38 grams

- Fats: 1 gram

- Fiber: 5 grams

- Sodium: 76 milligrams

- Protein: 5 grams

Poached Egg with Steamed Asparagus

Prep Time: 5 minutes
Cook Time: 10 minutes
Number of Servings: 2

Ingredients:

- 12 fresh asparagus spears

- 2 large eggs

- 1/2 teaspoon white vinegar

- Salt and pepper, to taste

- Chopped fresh parsley for garnish (optional)

Instructions:

1. Wash and trim the tough ends of 12 fresh asparagus spears.

2. In a wide saucepan, bring about 2 inches of water to a simmer. Add 1/2 teaspoon of white vinegar to the simmering water.

3. While the water is heating, prepare an ice bath in a bowl by filling it with ice and water.

4. Once the water is simmering, gently lower the asparagus spears into the saucepan. Steam them for about 3-4 minutes or until tender yet still crisp.

5. Use tongs to take out the steamed asparagus from the water and immediately plunge them into the ice bath to stop the cooking process. This helps the asparagus retain its vibrant green color and crispness. Drain and set aside.

6. In the same saucepan, add more water to a depth of about 2 inches and bring it to a gentle simmer again.

7. Crack 2 large eggs into separate small cups or ramekins.

8. Carefully slide each egg into the simmering water. Poach the eggs for about 3-4 minutes for runny yolks, or longer if you prefer them more well-done.

9. Use a slotted spoon to lift the poached eggs out of the water, allowing any excess water to drain.

10. Place 6 asparagus spears on each plate, and top them with a poached egg.

11. Season the dish with salt and pepper to taste.

12. If desired, garnish with chopped fresh parsley for added flavor and presentation.

13. Serve the poached egg with steamed asparagus immediately while warm.

Nutritional Information (per serving):

- Carbs: 5 grams

- Fats: 7 grams

- Fiber: 2 grams

- Sodium: 181 milligrams

- Protein: 8 grams

Blueberry Chia Pudding

Prep Time: 10 minutes
Cook Time: 0 minutes (Refrigeration time: 2-4 hours)
Number of Servings: 2

Ingredients:

- 1/2 cup fresh or frozen blueberries

- 1/4 cup chia seeds

- 1 cup lactose-free milk

- 1 tablespoon honey (optional)

- 1/4 teaspoon vanilla extract

Instructions:

1. If using frozen blueberries, allow them to thaw. If using fresh blueberries, you can skip this step.

2. In a blender or food processor, puree 1/2 cup of blueberries until smooth. You can add a little water if needed to achieve the desired consistency.

3. In a bowl, add the blueberry puree, 1/4 cup of chia seeds, one cup of lactose-free milk, one tablespoon of honey (if desired), and 1/4 teaspoon of vanilla extract.

4. Stir the mixture thoroughly to ensure that the chia seeds are well distributed.

5. Cover the bowl and refrigerate the blueberry chia pudding for at least 2-4 hours, or until it reaches the desired thickness. You can also leave it in the refrigerator overnight for a thicker consistency.

6. After the pudding has set, give it a good stir to fluff it up. If it's too thick, you can add a little more milk to reach your preferred consistency.

7. Divide the blueberry chia pudding into two serving glasses or bowls.

8. If desired, garnish with a few fresh blueberries.

9. Serve the pudding chilled.

Nutritional Information (per serving):

- Carbs: 27 grams

- Fats: 10 grams

- Fiber: 11 grams

- Sodium: 33 milligrams

- Protein: 6 grams

Sweet Potato Hash Browns

Prep Time: 15 minutes
Cook Time: 20 minutes
Number of Servings: 4

Ingredients:

- 2 medium sweet potatoes

- 2 tablespoons olive oil

- 1/2 onion, finely chopped

- 1/2 red bell pepper, diced

- 1/2 green bell pepper, diced

- Salt and pepper, to taste

- 1/2 teaspoon paprika (optional)

- Chopped fresh parsley for garnish (optional)

Instructions:

1. Peel and grate 2 medium sweet potatoes. Use a box grater or a food processor with a grating attachment for this.

2. Place the grated sweet potatoes in a clean kitchen towel or cheesecloth and squeeze out any excess moisture. This will help your hash browns crisp up better.

3. In a large skillet, heat two tablespoons of olive oil over medium heat.

4. Add 1/2 finely chopped onion and sauté for about 3 minutes, or until the onion becomes translucent.

5. Add the grated sweet potatoes to the skillet, spreading them out evenly.

6. Press down on the sweet potatoes with a spatula to create a compact layer. Let them cook without stirring for about 5-7 minutes, or until the bottom is golden brown and crispy.

7. Carefully flip the sweet potato hash browns to cook the other side. You can do this by sliding the hash browns onto a plate, then inverting them back into the skillet. Cook for another 5-7 minutes until the other side is crispy and golden.

8. While the hash browns are cooking, add 1/2 diced red bell pepper and 1/2 diced green bell pepper to the skillet. Sauté them alongside the hash browns until they become tender, about 3-4 minutes.

9. Season the hash browns and peppers with salt, pepper, and 1/2 teaspoon of paprika (if desired). Adjust the seasoning to your taste.

10. Once the sweet potato hash browns are cooked to your liking and the peppers are tender, take out the skillet from heat.

11. Garnish with chopped fresh parsley if desired.

12. Serve the sweet potato hash browns hot as a delicious side dish or breakfast item.

Nutritional Information (per serving):

- Carbs: 19 grams

- Fats: 7 grams
- Fiber: 3 grams
- Sodium: 176 milligrams
- Protein: 2 grams

SOUPS

Creamy Spinach and Potato Soup

Prep Time: 15 minutes
Cook Time: 30 minutes
Number of Servings: 4

Ingredients:

- 2 cups diced potatoes
- 4 cups low-sodium chicken broth
- 1 cup chopped spinach
- 1/2 cup finely diced onion
- 2 cloves minced garlic
- 1/2 cup heavy cream
- 2 tablespoons unsalted butter
- 1/2 teaspoon salt
- 1/4 teaspoon black pepper
- 1/4 teaspoon dried thyme
- 1/4 teaspoon dried rosemary
- 1/4 teaspoon dried oregano

Instructions:

1. In a large pot over medium heat, melt the butter. Add the diced onions and minced garlic, sautéing them until the onions become translucent, about 3-5 minutes.

2. Add the diced potatoes, chicken broth, salt, pepper, dried thyme, dried rosemary, and dried oregano to the pot. Bring the mixture to a boil, then reduce the heat to a simmer. Cover and cook for 15-20 minutes, or until the potatoes are tender.

3. Using an immersion blender or a regular blender, carefully puree the soup until it's smooth and creamy.

4. Return the pureed soup to the pot and stir in the chopped spinach. Simmer for an extra 5 minutes, or until the spinach is wilted.

5. Pour in the heavy cream, stirring until well combined. Heat the soup for an extra 2-3 minutes, ensuring not to bring it to a boil again.

6. Taste and adjust the seasoning, adding more salt and pepper if needed.

Nutritional Information (per serving):

- Carbs: 23g

- Fats: 15g

- Fiber: 3g

- Sodium: 480mg

- Protein: 4g

Cilantro Lime Chicken Soup

Prep Time: 15 minutes
Cook Time: 25 minutes
Number of Servings: 4

Ingredients:

- 2 boneless, skinless chicken breasts, diced into small pieces

- 6 cups low-sodium chicken broth

- 1 cup diced carrots

- 1 cup diced celery

- 1/2 cup finely chopped onion

- 2 cloves garlic, minced

- 1/4 cup fresh cilantro leaves, chopped

- Juice of 2 limes

- 1/2 teaspoon salt

- 1/4 teaspoon black pepper

- 1/4 teaspoon dried oregano

Instructions:

1. In a large pot, add the diced chicken, chicken broth, diced carrots, diced celery, finely chopped onion, minced garlic, salt, black pepper, and dried oregano.

2. Bring the mixture to a boil over medium-high heat. Once boiling, reduce the heat to a simmer and cover the pot. Cook for 15-20 minutes, or until the chicken is properly cooked and the vegetables are tender.

3. Stir in the chopped cilantro and lime juice. Simmer for an extra 5 minutes to allow the flavors to meld.

4. Taste and adjust the seasoning, adding more salt and pepper if desired.

Nutritional Information (per serving):

- Carbs: 8g

- Fats: 2g

- Fiber: 1g

- Sodium: 320mg

- Protein: 22g

Roasted Red Pepper and Tomato Bisque

Prep Time: 15 minutes
Cook Time: 35 minutes
Number of Servings: 4

Ingredients:

- 2 red bell peppers, roasted, peeled, and diced

- 2 large tomatoes, diced

- 1/2 cup diced onion

- 2 cloves garlic, minced

- 4 cups low-sodium chicken broth

- 1/2 cup heavy cream

- 2 tablespoons olive oil

- 1/2 teaspoon salt

- 1/4 teaspoon black pepper

- 1/4 teaspoon dried basil

- 1/4 teaspoon dried thyme

- 1/4 teaspoon dried oregano

Instructions:

1. Start by roasting the red bell peppers. Turn on your oven and set it to 450°F (230°C). Place the whole peppers on a baking sheet and roast them for about 20-25 minutes, turning occasionally, until the skins are charred and blistered. Take it out from the oven, place them in a bowl, and cover with plastic wrap for 10 minutes. This will make it easier to peel them. After 10 minutes, peel, seed, and dice the roasted peppers.

2. In a large pot, heat the olive oil over medium heat. Add the diced onions and minced garlic. Sauté until the onions are translucent, about 3-5 minutes.

3. Add the diced tomatoes, roasted red peppers, chicken broth, salt, black pepper, dried basil, dried thyme, and dried oregano to the pot. Bring the mixture to a boil, then reduce the heat to a simmer. Cover and cook for 15-20 minutes, allowing the flavors to meld.

4. Using an immersion blender or a regular blender, carefully puree the soup until it's smooth.

5. Return the pureed soup to the pot and stir in the heavy cream. Heat the soup over low heat for an extra 5 minutes, ensuring not to bring it to a boil.

6. Taste and adjust the seasoning, adding more salt and pepper if needed.

Nutritional Information (per serving):

- Carbs: 12g

- Fats: 12g

- Fiber: 2g

- Sodium: 420mg

- Protein: 5g

Shrimp and Quinoa Chowder

Prep Time: 15 minutes
Cook Time: 30 minutes
Number of Servings: 4

Ingredients:

- 1 cup cooked quinoa

- 1 pound large shrimp, peeled and deveined

- 4 cups low-sodium chicken broth

- 1 cup diced carrots

- 1 cup diced celery

- 1/2 cup finely chopped onion

- 2 cloves garlic, minced

- 1/2 cup unsalted butter

- 1/2 cup whole milk

- 1/2 teaspoon salt

- 1/4 teaspoon black pepper

- 1/4 teaspoon dried thyme

- 1/4 teaspoon dried rosemary

- 1/4 teaspoon dried oregano

Instructions:

1. In a large pot, melt the unsalted butter over medium heat. Add the diced onions and minced garlic, sautéing them until the onions become translucent, about 3-5 minutes.

2. Add the diced carrots, diced celery, salt, black pepper, dried thyme, dried rosemary, and dried oregano to the pot. Sauté for an extra 5 minutes, until the vegetables begin to soften.

3. Pour in the low-sodium chicken broth and bring the mixture to a boil. Reduce the heat to a simmer and cover the pot. Cook for 15-20 minutes, or until the carrots and celery are tender.

4. Stir in the cooked quinoa and whole milk, allowing the soup to simmer for an extra 5 minutes.

5. While the soup is simmering, cook the peeled and deveined shrimp in a separate pan over medium heat until they turn pink, about 2-3 minutes per side.

6. Divide the cooked shrimp among the serving bowls.

7. Ladle the hot quinoa and vegetable chowder over the cooked shrimp in each bowl.

Nutritional Information (per serving):

- Carbs: 31g

- Fats: 22g

- Fiber: 4g

- Sodium: 460mg

- Protein: 29g

Creamy Parsnip and Apple Soup

Prep Time: 15 minutes
Cook Time: 30 minutes
Number of Servings: 4

Ingredients:

- 4 cups diced parsnips

- 2 cups diced apples (peeled and cored)

- 1 cup chopped leeks (white and light green parts only)
- 2 cloves garlic, minced
- 4 cups low-sodium vegetable broth
- 1/2 cup whole milk
- 2 tablespoons unsalted butter
- 2 tablespoons olive oil
- 1/2 teaspoon salt
- 1/4 teaspoon black pepper
- 1/4 teaspoon dried thyme
- 1/4 teaspoon dried rosemary
- 1/4 teaspoon dried sage

Instructions:

1. In a large pot, heat the olive oil and unsalted butter over medium heat. Add the chopped leeks and minced garlic, sautéing them until the leeks become soft and translucent, about 3-5 minutes.

2. Add the diced parsnips, diced apples, salt, black pepper, dried thyme, dried rosemary, and dried sage to the pot. Continue to sauté for an extra 5 minutes to allow the flavors to meld.

3. Pour in the low-sodium vegetable broth and bring the mixture to a boil. Reduce the heat to a simmer, cover the pot, and cook for 15-20 minutes, or until the parsnips and apples are tender.

4. Using an immersion blender or a regular blender, carefully puree the soup until it's smooth and creamy.

5. Return the pureed soup to the pot and stir in the whole milk. Heat the soup over low heat for an extra 5 minutes, ensuring not to bring it to a boil again.

6. Taste and adjust the seasoning, adding more salt and pepper if needed.

Nutritional Information (per serving):

- Carbs: 37g

- Fats: 14g

- Fiber: 8g

- Sodium: 480mg

- Protein: 4g

Lemon Chicken and Rice Soup

Prep Time: 15 minutes
Cook Time: 35 minutes
Number of Servings: 4

Ingredients:

- 2 boneless, skinless chicken breasts, diced into small pieces

- 1 cup long-grain white rice

- 6 cups low-sodium chicken broth

- 1/2 cup diced carrots

- 1/2 cup diced celery

- 1/2 cup finely chopped onion

- 2 cloves garlic, minced

- Juice of 2 lemons

- Zest of 1 lemon

- 1/2 teaspoon salt

- 1/4 teaspoon black pepper

- 1/4 teaspoon dried thyme

- 1/4 teaspoon dried rosemary

- 1/4 teaspoon dried oregano

Instructions:

1. In a large pot, add the diced chicken, white rice, low-sodium chicken broth, diced carrots, diced celery, finely chopped onion,

minced garlic, salt, black pepper, dried thyme, dried rosemary, and dried oregano.

2. Bring the mixture to a boil over medium-high heat. Once boiling, reduce the heat to a simmer. Cover the pot and cook for 15-20 minutes, or until the chicken is properly cooked, and the rice and vegetables are tender.

3. Stir in the lemon juice and lemon zest, allowing the soup to simmer for an extra 5 minutes to incorporate the lemony flavor.

4. Taste and adjust the seasoning, adding more salt and pepper if desired.

Nutritional Information (per serving):

- Carbs: 36g

- Fats: 3g

- Fiber: 2g

- Sodium: 420mg

- Protein: 18g

White Bean and Kale Soup

Prep Time: 15 minutes
Cook Time: 30 minutes
Number of Servings: 4

Ingredients:

- 2 cups canned white beans (such as cannellini or navy beans), drained and rinsed

- 4 cups low-sodium vegetable broth

- 2 cups chopped kale, stems removed

- 1 cup diced carrots

- 1 cup diced celery

- 1/2 cup finely chopped onion

- 2 cloves garlic, minced

- 2 tablespoons olive oil
- 1/2 teaspoon salt
- 1/4 teaspoon black pepper
- 1/4 teaspoon dried thyme
- 1/4 teaspoon dried rosemary
- 1/4 teaspoon dried oregano

Instructions:

1. In a large pot, heat the olive oil over medium heat. Add the diced onions and minced garlic, sautéing them until the onions become translucent, about 3-5 minutes.

2. Add the diced carrots, diced celery, salt, black pepper, dried thyme, dried rosemary, and dried oregano to the pot. Sauté for an extra 5 minutes to soften the vegetables.

3. Pour in the low-sodium vegetable broth and bring the mixture to a boil. Reduce the heat to a simmer, cover the pot, and cook for 15-20 minutes, or until the vegetables are tender.

4. Add the canned white beans to the pot and continue to simmer for an extra 5 minutes.

5. Stir in the chopped kale and cook for an extra 5 minutes, or until the kale is wilted and tender.

6. Taste and adjust the seasoning, adding more salt and pepper if needed.

Nutritional Information (per serving):

- Carbs: 34g
- Fats: 7g
- Fiber: 8g
- Sodium: 420mg
- Protein: 9g

Creamy Mushroom and Rice Soup

Prep Time: 15 minutes
Cook Time: 30 minutes
Number of Servings: 4

Ingredients:

- 2 cups sliced mushrooms
- 1 cup cooked white rice
- 4 cups low-sodium vegetable broth
- 1/2 cup chopped leeks (white and light green parts only)
- 1/2 cup finely chopped onion
- 2 cloves garlic, minced
- 1/2 cup heavy cream
- 2 tablespoons unsalted butter
- 2 tablespoons olive oil
- 1/2 teaspoon salt
- 1/4 teaspoon black pepper
- 1/4 teaspoon dried thyme
- 1/4 teaspoon dried rosemary
- 1/4 teaspoon dried oregano

Instructions:

1. In a large pot, heat the olive oil and unsalted butter over medium heat. Add the chopped leeks and minced garlic, sautéing them until the leeks become soft and translucent, about 3-5 minutes.

2. Add the sliced mushrooms, finely chopped onion, salt, black pepper, dried thyme, dried rosemary, and dried oregano to the pot. Continue to sauté for an extra 5 minutes, until the mushrooms are tender and the onions are translucent.

3. Pour in the low-sodium vegetable broth and bring the mixture to a boil. Reduce the heat to a simmer, cover the pot, and cook for 15-20 minutes, allowing the flavors to meld.

4. Stir in the cooked white rice and heavy cream, allowing the soup to simmer for an extra 5 minutes to heat through.

5. Taste and adjust the seasoning, adding more salt and pepper if needed.

Nutritional Information (per serving):

- Carbs: 24g

- Fats: 16g

- Fiber: 2g

- Sodium: 480mg

- Protein: 4g

Sweet Potato and Leek Soup

Prep Time: 15 minutes
Cook Time: 30 minutes
Number of Servings: 4

Ingredients:

- 2 cups diced sweet potatoes

- 2 cups chopped leeks (white and light green parts only)

- 4 cups low-sodium vegetable broth

- 1/2 cup whole milk

- 2 tablespoons unsalted butter

- 2 tablespoons olive oil

- 1/2 teaspoon salt

- 1/4 teaspoon black pepper

- 1/4 teaspoon dried thyme

- 1/4 teaspoon dried rosemary

- 1/4 teaspoon dried sage

Instructions:

1. In a large pot, heat the olive oil and unsalted butter over medium heat. Add the chopped leeks and sauté until they become soft and translucent, about 3-5 minutes.

2. Add the diced sweet potatoes, salt, black pepper, dried thyme, dried rosemary, and dried sage to the pot. Continue to sauté for an extra 5 minutes to infuse the flavors.

3. Pour in the low-sodium vegetable broth and bring the mixture to a boil. Reduce the heat to a simmer, cover the pot, and cook for 15-20 minutes, or until the sweet potatoes are tender.

4. Using an immersion blender or a regular blender, carefully puree the soup until it's smooth.

5. Return the pureed soup to the pot and stir in the whole milk. Heat the soup over low heat for an extra 5 minutes, ensuring not to bring it to a boil.

6. Taste and adjust the seasoning, adding more salt and pepper if needed.

Nutritional Information (per serving):

- Carbs: 22g

- Fats: 11g

- Fiber: 3g

- Sodium: 480mg

- Protein: 4g

Turkey Meatball Soup with Rice

Prep Time: 20 minutes
Cook Time: 30 minutes
Number of Servings: 4

Ingredients:

For Turkey Meatballs:

- 1/2 pound ground turkey
- 1/4 cup breadcrumbs
- 1/4 cup grated Parmesan cheese
- 1/4 cup finely chopped fresh parsley
- 1/4 teaspoon salt
- 1/4 teaspoon black pepper
- 1/4 teaspoon dried oregano
- 1/4 teaspoon dried basil
- 1/4 teaspoon dried thyme

For Soup:

- 4 cups low-sodium chicken broth
- 1 cup cooked white rice
- 1/2 cup diced carrots
- 1/2 cup diced celery
- 1/2 cup finely chopped onion
- 2 cloves garlic, minced
- 2 tablespoons olive oil
- 1/2 teaspoon salt
- 1/4 teaspoon black pepper
- 1/4 teaspoon dried thyme
- 1/4 teaspoon dried rosemary

Instructions:

For Turkey Meatballs:

1. In a mixing bowl, add the ground turkey, breadcrumbs, grated Parmesan cheese, finely chopped fresh parsley, salt, black pepper, dried oregano, dried basil, and dried thyme. Mix sufficiently.

2. Form the mixture into small meatballs, about 1 inch in diameter.

For Soup:

1. In a large pot, heat the olive oil over medium heat. Add the diced onions and minced garlic, sautéing them until the onions become translucent, about 3-5 minutes.

2. Add the diced carrots, diced celery, salt, black pepper, dried thyme, and dried rosemary to the pot. Sauté for an extra 5 minutes to soften the vegetables.

3. Pour in the low-sodium chicken broth and bring the mixture to a boil. Reduce the heat to a simmer, cover the pot, and cook for 15-20 minutes, allowing the flavors to meld.

4. Carefully drop the turkey meatballs into the simmering soup. Cook for 10-15 minutes, or until the meatballs are properly cooked.

5. Stir in the cooked white rice and heat for an extra 5 minutes to warm the rice.

6. Taste and adjust the seasoning, adding more salt and pepper if needed.

Nutritional Information (per serving):

- Carbs: 32g

- Fats: 9g

- Fiber: 2g

- Sodium: 480mg

- Protein: 20g

Butternut Squash Soup with Ginger

Prep Time: 15 minutes
Cook Time: 35 minutes
Number of Servings: 4

Ingredients:

- 4 cups peeled, seeded, and cubed butternut squash

- 1 cup diced onion
- 1/2 cup chopped carrot
- 1/2 cup chopped celery
- 2 cloves garlic, minced
- 1 tablespoon freshly grated ginger
- 4 cups low-sodium vegetable broth
- 1/2 cup whole milk
- 2 tablespoons unsalted butter
- 2 tablespoons olive oil
- 1/2 teaspoon salt
- 1/4 teaspoon black pepper
- 1/4 teaspoon ground cinnamon
- 1/4 teaspoon ground nutmeg

Instructions:

1. In a large pot, heat the olive oil and unsalted butter over medium heat. Add the diced onions, chopped carrots, chopped celery, minced garlic, and freshly grated ginger. Sauté them until the vegetables become soft and the onions are translucent, about 5-7 minutes.

2. Add the peeled, seeded, and cubed butternut squash to the pot, along with the salt, black pepper, ground cinnamon, and ground nutmeg. Sauté for an extra 5 minutes to coat the squash with the spices.

3. Pour in the low-sodium vegetable broth and bring the mixture to a boil. Reduce the heat to a simmer, cover the pot, and cook for 15-20 minutes, or until the butternut squash is tender.

4. Using an immersion blender or a regular blender, carefully puree the soup until it's smooth.

5. Return the pureed soup to the pot and stir in the whole milk. Heat the soup over low heat for an extra 5 minutes, ensuring not to bring it to a boil again.

6. Taste and adjust the seasoning, adding more salt and pepper if needed.

Nutritional Information (per serving):

- Carbs: 29g

- Fats: 10g

- Fiber: 6g

- Sodium: 680mg

- Protein: 3g

Chicken and Rice Congee

Prep Time: 15 minutes
Cook Time: 1 hour 30 minutes
Number of Servings: 4

Ingredients:

- 1 cup white rice

- 4 cups low-sodium chicken broth

- 2 cups water

- 1 cup cooked and shredded chicken breast

- 1/2 cup finely chopped carrots

- 1/2 cup finely chopped celery

- 1/2 cup finely chopped zucchini

- 1/4 cup finely chopped green onions

- 2 cloves garlic, minced

- 1 tablespoon ginger, minced

- 1 tablespoon vegetable oil

- 1/2 teaspoon salt

- 1/4 teaspoon black pepper

- 1/4 teaspoon dried thyme

Instructions:

1. Rinse the white rice under cold water until the water runs clear. Drain well.

2. In a large pot, heat the vegetable oil over medium heat. Add the minced garlic and ginger, and sauté for about 1-2 minutes until fragrant.

3. Add the rinsed rice to the pot and stir, allowing it to toast for about 2-3 minutes.

4. Pour in the low-sodium chicken broth and water. Bring the mixture to a boil, then reduce the heat to a low simmer.

5. Cover the pot partially and simmer the rice for 1 hour, stirring occasionally. The rice will break down and thicken the congee.

6. After 1 hour, add the cooked and shredded chicken, finely chopped carrots, celery, zucchini, green onions, salt, black pepper, and dried thyme to the pot.

7. Continue to simmer for an extra 15-20 minutes, or until the vegetables are tender and the congee has reached your desired consistency.

8. Taste and adjust the seasoning, adding more salt and pepper if needed.

Nutritional Information (per serving):

- Carbs: 48g

- Fats: 6g

- Fiber: 3g

- Sodium: 580mg

- Protein: 16g

Creamy Tomato Soup with Rice

Prep Time: 15 minutes
Cook Time: 30 minutes
Number of Servings: 4

Ingredients:

- 2 cups canned tomato puree
- 1/2 cup cooked white rice
- 4 cups low-sodium vegetable broth
- 1/2 cup whole milk
- 2 tablespoons unsalted butter
- 2 tablespoons olive oil
- 1/2 cup finely chopped onion
- 2 cloves garlic, minced
- 1/2 teaspoon salt
- 1/4 teaspoon black pepper
- 1/4 teaspoon dried basil
- 1/4 teaspoon dried oregano
- 1/4 teaspoon dried thyme

Instructions:

1. In a large pot, heat the olive oil and unsalted butter over medium heat. Add the finely chopped onions and minced garlic, sautéing them until the onions become soft and translucent, about 3-5 minutes.

2. Add the canned tomato puree, salt, black pepper, dried basil, dried oregano, and dried thyme to the pot. Stir to combine and cook for an extra 5 minutes to allow the flavors to meld.

3. Pour in the low-sodium vegetable broth and bring the mixture to a boil. Reduce the heat to a simmer, cover the pot, and cook for 15-20 minutes, allowing the soup to thicken and the flavors to develop.

4. Stir in the cooked white rice and whole milk, allowing the soup to simmer for an extra 5 minutes to heat through.

5. Taste and adjust the seasoning, adding more salt and pepper if needed.

Nutritional Information (per serving):

- Carbs: 33g

- Fats: 12g

- Fiber: 4g

- Sodium: 780mg

- Protein: 6g

Miso Soup with Silken Tofu

Prep Time: 10 minutes
Cook Time: 10 minutes
Number of Servings: 4

Ingredients:

- 4 cups low-sodium vegetable broth

- 1/2 cup miso paste

- 8 ounces silken tofu, diced into small cubes

- 1/2 cup sliced green onions

- 1/2 cup sliced mushrooms (shiitake or white mushrooms)

- 2 sheets nori (seaweed), cut into thin strips

- 1 tablespoon vegetable oil

- 1 teaspoon sesame oil

- 1/4 teaspoon salt

- 1/4 teaspoon black pepper

Instructions:

1. In a pot, heat the vegetable oil over medium heat. Add the sliced mushrooms and sauté them for about 3-5 minutes, or until they start to soften.

2. Pour in the low-sodium vegetable broth and bring it to a gentle simmer.

3. In a small bowl, whisk the miso paste with a ladleful of hot broth until it's well combined and smooth.

4. Gradually add the miso mixture back into the pot, stirring well to fully incorporate it into the broth.

5. Add the diced silken tofu and sliced green onions to the pot. Continue to simmer for another 2-3 minutes, allowing the tofu to heat through.

6. Stir in the sesame oil, salt, and black pepper. Taste and adjust the seasoning, adding more salt or pepper if needed.

7. To serve, ladle the hot miso soup into bowls and garnish with nori strips.

Nutritional Information (per serving):

- Carbs: 10g

- Fats: 4g

- Fiber: 2g

- Sodium: 760mg

- Protein: 7g

Potato Leek Soup with a Hint of Nutmeg

Prep Time: 15 minutes
Cook Time: 30 minutes
Number of Servings: 4

Ingredients:

- 4 cups diced potatoes

- 2 cups chopped leeks (white and light green parts only)

- 4 cups low-sodium vegetable broth

- 1/2 cup whole milk

- 2 tablespoons unsalted butter

- 2 tablespoons olive oil

- 1/2 teaspoon salt

- 1/4 teaspoon black pepper

- 1/4 teaspoon ground nutmeg

- 1/4 teaspoon dried thyme

Instructions:

1. In a large pot, heat the olive oil and unsalted butter over medium heat. Add the chopped leeks and sauté until they become soft and translucent, about 3-5 minutes.

2. Add the diced potatoes, salt, black pepper, ground nutmeg, and dried thyme to the pot. Continue to sauté for an extra 5 minutes to infuse the flavors.

3. Pour in the low-sodium vegetable broth and bring the mixture to a boil. Reduce the heat to a simmer, cover the pot, and cook for 15-20 minutes, or until the potatoes are tender.

4. Using an immersion blender or a regular blender, carefully puree the soup until it's smooth.

5. Return the pureed soup to the pot and stir in the whole milk. Heat the soup over low heat for an extra 5 minutes, ensuring not to bring it to a boil again.

6. Taste and adjust the seasoning, adding more salt and pepper if needed.

Nutritional Information (per serving):

- Carbs: 32g

- Fats: 9g

- Fiber: 4g

- Sodium: 720mg

- Protein: 4g

Lentil and Spinach Stew

Prep Time: 15 minutes
Cook Time: 45 minutes
Number of Servings: 4

Ingredients:

- 1 cup dried green or brown lentils
- 4 cups low-sodium vegetable broth
- 2 cups chopped spinach
- 1 cup diced carrots
- 1 cup diced celery
- 1/2 cup finely chopped onion
- 2 cloves garlic, minced
- 2 tablespoons olive oil
- 1/2 teaspoon salt
- 1/4 teaspoon black pepper
- 1/4 teaspoon dried thyme
- 1/4 teaspoon dried rosemary

Instructions:

1. In a large pot, heat the olive oil over medium heat. Add the finely chopped onions and minced garlic, sautéing them until the onions become soft and translucent, about 3-5 minutes.

2. Add the diced carrots, diced celery, salt, black pepper, dried thyme, and dried rosemary to the pot. Continue to sauté for an extra 5 minutes to soften the vegetables.

3. Rinse the dried lentils under cold water and drain well. Add them to the pot.

4. Pour in the low-sodium vegetable broth and bring the mixture to a boil. Reduce the heat to a simmer, cover the pot, and cook for 30-35 minutes, or until the lentils are tender.

5. Stir in the chopped spinach and cook for an extra 5 minutes, or until the spinach is wilted.

6. Taste and adjust the seasoning, adding more salt and pepper if needed.

Nutritional Information (per serving):

- Carbs: 41g

- Fats: 7g

- Fiber: 16g

- Sodium: 760mg

- Protein: 16g

Turkey and Vegetable Broth

Prep Time: 15 minutes
Cook Time: 2 hours
Number of Servings: 6

Ingredients:

- 1 pound turkey breast, bone-in and skin-on

- 8 cups water

- 2 cups diced carrots

- 2 cups diced celery

- 1 cup diced onion

- 2 cloves garlic, minced

- 1 bay leaf

- 1/2 teaspoon salt

- 1/4 teaspoon black pepper

- 1/4 teaspoon dried thyme

- 1/4 teaspoon dried rosemary

Instructions:

1. In a large pot, place the turkey breast, bone-in and skin-on, and cover it with 8 cups of water.

2. Bring the water to a boil, then reduce the heat to a simmer. Allow the turkey to simmer for 1 hour, skimming any foam that forms on the surface.

3. After 1 hour, take out the turkey breast from the pot and set it aside to cool. Once cooled, shred the turkey meat into bite-sized pieces, discarding the skin and bones.

4. Return the shredded turkey meat to the pot of broth.

5. Add the diced carrots, diced celery, diced onion, minced garlic, bay leaf, salt, black pepper, dried thyme, and dried rosemary to the pot with the turkey and broth.

6. Continue to simmer the mixture for an extra 30 minutes to 1 hour, or until the vegetables are tender and the flavors meld together.

7. Taste and adjust the seasoning, adding more salt and pepper if needed.

Nutritional Information (per serving):

- Carbs: 6g

- Fats: 1g

- Fiber: 2g

- Sodium: 420mg

- Protein: 25g

Creamy Cauliflower Soup

Prep Time: 15 minutes
Cook Time: 30 minutes
Number of Servings: 4

Ingredients:

- 1 large head of cauliflower, cut into florets

- 4 cups low-sodium vegetable broth

- 1 cup whole milk
- 2 tablespoons unsalted butter
- 2 tablespoons olive oil
- 1/2 cup finely chopped onion
- 2 cloves garlic, minced
- 1/2 teaspoon salt
- 1/4 teaspoon black pepper
- 1/4 teaspoon dried thyme
- 1/4 teaspoon dried rosemary

Instructions:

1. In a large pot, heat the olive oil and unsalted butter over medium heat. Add the finely chopped onions and minced garlic, sautéing them until the onions become soft and translucent, about 3-5 minutes.

2. Add the cauliflower florets, salt, black pepper, dried thyme, and dried rosemary to the pot. Continue to sauté for an extra 5 minutes to infuse the flavors.

3. Pour in the low-sodium vegetable broth and bring the mixture to a boil. Reduce the heat to a simmer, cover the pot, and cook for 15-20 minutes, or until the cauliflower is tender.

4. Using an immersion blender or a regular blender, carefully puree the soup until it's smooth.

5. Return the pureed soup to the pot and stir in the whole milk. Heat the soup over low heat for an extra 5 minutes, ensuring not to bring it to a boil again.

6. Taste and adjust the seasoning, adding more salt and pepper if needed.

Nutritional Information (per serving):

- Carbs: 15g
- Fats: 10g

- Fiber: 4g
- Sodium: 480mg
- Protein: 5g

- Fiber: 4g
- Sodium: 480mg
- Protein: 5g

SALADS

Spinach and Quinoa Salad with Lemon Dressing

Prep Time: 15 minutes
Cook Time: 15 minutes
Number of Servings: 4

Ingredients:

For the Salad:

- 2 cups fresh spinach leaves, washed and chopped
- 1 cup cooked quinoa, cooled
- 1 cup diced cucumber
- 1 cup diced red bell pepper
- 1/2 cup diced red onion
- 1/4 cup crumbled feta cheese (optional)

For the Lemon Dressing:

- 1/4 cup fresh lemon juice
- 1/4 cup olive oil
- 2 teaspoons honey
- 1 clove garlic, minced
- Salt and pepper to taste

Instructions:

1. In a large salad bowl, add the fresh spinach leaves, cooked and cooled quinoa, diced cucumber, diced red bell pepper, and diced red onion.

2. If you're following a gastroparesis diet, ensure all ingredients are well-cooked and soft to avoid digestive issues.

3. In a separate small bowl, prepare the Lemon Dressing. Whisk the fresh lemon juice, olive oil, honey, minced garlic, and season with a pinch of salt and pepper. Mix until well combined.

4. Pour the Lemon Dressing over the salad mixture.

5. Gently toss the salad to coat all the ingredients evenly with the dressing.

6. If desired, sprinkle the crumbled feta cheese over the top of the salad for added flavor. (Note: Skip this step if dairy is not suitable for your gastroparesis diet.)

7. Serve the Spinach and Quinoa Salad immediately or refrigerate for later use. The salad can be enjoyed cold or at room temperature.

Nutritional Information (per serving):

- Carbohydrates: 33g
- Fats: 14g
- Fiber: 5g
- Sodium: 180mg
- Protein: 7g

Shredded Carrot and Apple Salad

Prep Time: 15 minutes
Cook Time: 0 minutes
Number of Servings: 4

Ingredients:

For the Salad:

- 2 cups shredded carrots
- 2 cups shredded apples (use a sweet variety like Gala or Fuji)
- 1/2 cup finely chopped pecans or walnuts (optional, omit if needed)
- 1/4 cup dried cranberries (optional, omit if needed)

For the Dressing:

- 2 tablespoons olive oil
- 2 tablespoons apple cider vinegar

- 1 tablespoon honey
- 1/2 teaspoon ground cinnamon
- A pinch of salt

Instructions:

1. In a large bowl, add the shredded carrots and shredded apples.

2. If you're following a gastroparesis diet, make sure the carrots and apples are finely shredded to aid in digestion.

3. If using, add the finely chopped pecans or walnuts to the bowl. (Note: Skip this step if nuts are not suitable for your gastroparesis diet.)

4. If using, add the dried cranberries to the bowl. (Note: Skip this step if dried fruits are not suitable for your gastroparesis diet.)

5. In a separate small bowl, prepare the dressing. Whisk the olive oil, apple cider vinegar, honey, ground cinnamon, and a pinch of salt until well combined.

6. Pour the dressing over the salad mixture.

7. Gently toss the salad to ensure all ingredients are coated with the dressing.

8. Serve the Shredded Carrot and Apple Salad immediately, or refrigerate it for later use. This salad can be enjoyed chilled.

Nutritional Information (per serving):

- Carbohydrates: 27g
- Fats: 9g
- Fiber: 4g
- Sodium: 74mg
- Protein: 1g

Tofu and Broccoli Slaw Salad

Prep Time: 20 minutes
Cook Time: 10 minutes
Number of Servings: 4

Ingredients:

For the Salad:

- 1 block (14 ounces) extra-firm tofu, pressed and cubed
- 4 cups broccoli slaw mix (shredded broccoli stems and carrots)
- 1/2 cup thinly sliced red cabbage
- 1/4 cup chopped green onions
- 1/4 cup chopped fresh cilantro

For the Dressing:

- 3 tablespoons rice vinegar
- 2 tablespoons low-sodium soy sauce
- 1 tablespoon sesame oil
- 1 tablespoon honey
- 1 clove garlic, minced
- 1/2 teaspoon grated fresh ginger
- A pinch of salt

Instructions:

1. Begin by pressing the tofu to remove excess moisture. To do this, place the tofu block on a plate, top it with another plate, and weigh it down with a heavy object (like a can or skillet). Press for at least 15 minutes, then cube the tofu into bite-sized pieces.

2. In a large bowl, add the broccoli slaw mix, thinly sliced red cabbage, chopped green onions, and chopped fresh cilantro.

3. If you're following a gastroparesis diet, make sure the broccoli slaw is finely shredded to aid in digestion.

4. In a separate small bowl, prepare the dressing. Whisk the rice vinegar, low-sodium soy sauce, sesame oil, honey, minced garlic, grated fresh ginger, and a pinch of salt until well combined.

5. Heat a non-stick skillet over medium heat. Add the cubed tofu and cook until it's lightly browned on all sides, about 5-7 minutes. You can use a small amount of oil if needed, but avoid excess oil if it's not suitable for your gastroparesis diet.

6. Once the tofu is cooked, remove it from the skillet and let it cool slightly.

7. Add the cooked tofu to the salad mixture.

8. Pour the dressing over the salad and tofu.

9. Gently toss the salad to ensure all ingredients are coated with the dressing.

10. Serve the Tofu and Broccoli Slaw Salad immediately, or refrigerate for later use. This salad can be enjoyed cold or at room temperature.

Nutritional Information (per serving):

- Carbohydrates: 17g

- Fats: 10g

- Fiber: 5g

- Sodium: 437mg

- Protein: 11g

Pear and Walnut Salad

Prep Time: 15 minutes
Cook Time: 0 minutes
Number of Servings: 4

Ingredients:

For the Salad:

- 4 cups mixed salad greens (e.g., lettuce, spinach, arugula)

- 2 ripe pears, thinly sliced
- 1/2 cup chopped walnuts
- 1/4 cup crumbled blue cheese (optional, omit if needed)

For the Dressing:

- 2 tablespoons extra-virgin olive oil
- 2 tablespoons balsamic vinegar
- 1 tablespoon honey
- A pinch of salt

Instructions:

1. In a large bowl, add the mixed salad greens.

2. If you're following a gastroparesis diet, ensure the salad greens are well-washed and free of tough stems.

3. Thinly slice the ripe pears and add them to the salad greens.

4. If using, sprinkle the chopped walnuts over the salad. (Note: Skip this step if nuts are not suitable for your gastroparesis diet.)

5. If using, crumble the blue cheese over the salad. (Note: Skip this step if dairy is not suitable for your gastroparesis diet.)

6. In a separate small bowl, prepare the dressing. Whisk the extra-virgin olive oil, balsamic vinegar, honey, and a pinch of salt until well combined.

7. Drizzle the dressing over the salad mixture.

8. Gently toss the salad to ensure all ingredients are coated with the dressing.

9. Serve the Pear and Walnut Salad immediately, ensuring it's at a comfortable temperature for your diet.

Nutritional Information (per serving):

- Carbohydrates: 27g
- Fats: 18g
- Fiber: 5g

- Sodium: 193mg

- Protein: 4g

Roasted Beet and Arugula Salad

Prep Time: 15 minutes
Cook Time: 45 minutes
Number of Servings: 4

Ingredients:

For the Salad:

- 4 medium-sized beets, peeled and diced into 1/2-inch cubes

- 8 cups fresh arugula leaves, washed and dried

- 1/2 cup crumbled goat cheese (optional, omit if needed)

- 1/4 cup chopped walnuts (optional, omit if needed)

For the Dressing:

- 3 tablespoons extra-virgin olive oil

- 2 tablespoons balsamic vinegar

- 1 teaspoon honey

- A pinch of salt and pepper

Instructions:

1. Turn on your oven and set it to 400°F (200°C).

2. In a baking dish, place the diced beets. Drizzle with one tablespoon of extra-virgin olive oil and season with a pinch of salt and pepper. Toss to coat evenly.

3. Roast the beets in the preheated oven for about 45 minutes or until tender and can be easily pierced with a fork.

4. While the beets are roasting, prepare the dressing. In a small bowl, whisk two tablespoons of balsamic vinegar, two tablespoons of extra-virgin olive oil, one teaspoon of honey, and a pinch of salt and pepper. Set the dressing aside.

5. Once the beets are roasted and tender, take them out from the oven and allow them to cool for a few minutes.

6. In a large salad bowl, place the washed and dried arugula leaves.

7. If you're following a gastroparesis diet, ensure that the arugula leaves are well-washed and free of any tough stems.

8. Add the roasted beets to the arugula.

9. If using, sprinkle the crumbled goat cheese over the salad. (Note: Skip this step if dairy is not suitable for your gastroparesis diet.)

10. If using, scatter the chopped walnuts over the salad. (Note: Skip this step if nuts are not suitable for your gastroparesis diet.)

11. Drizzle the prepared dressing over the salad.

12. Gently toss the salad to ensure all ingredients are coated with the dressing.

13. Serve the Roasted Beet and Arugula Salad immediately while the beets are still warm or at a temperature suitable for your diet.

Nutritional Information (per serving):

- Carbohydrates: 15g

- Fats: 14g

- Fiber: 3g

- Sodium: 135mg

- Protein: 6g

Grape and Cottage Cheese Salad

Prep Time: 10 minutes
Cook Time: 0 minutes
Number of Servings: 2

Ingredients:

For the Salad:

- 2 cups seedless grapes, halved

- 1 cup low-fat cottage cheese

- 1/4 cup chopped fresh mint leaves

For the Dressing:

- 1 tablespoon honey

- 1 tablespoon lemon juice

- A pinch of salt

Instructions:

1. In a bowl, add the halved seedless grapes.

2. If you're following a gastroparesis diet, make sure the grapes are well-washed, and you can remove any stems or tough skin if necessary.

3. In a separate bowl, place the low-fat cottage cheese.

4. If you're following a gastroparesis diet, choose a cottage cheese variety that is easy to digest.

5. Chop the fresh mint leaves finely.

6. Add the chopped fresh mint leaves to the cottage cheese.

7. In a small bowl, prepare the dressing by whisking together one tablespoon of honey, one tablespoon of lemon juice, and a pinch of salt.

8. Pour the dressing over the cottage cheese and mint mixture.

9. Gently stir the cottage cheese mixture to incorporate the dressing.

10. Divide the dressed cottage cheese mixture between two serving plates.

11. Top each serving with the halved grapes.

12. Serve the Grape and Cottage Cheese Salad immediately at a temperature suitable for your diet.

Nutritional Information (per serving):

- Carbohydrates: 34g

- Fats: 2g

- Fiber: 2g

- Sodium: 446mg

- Protein: 16g

Caprese Salad with Balsamic Glaze

Prep Time: 10 minutes
Cook Time: 0 minutes
Number of Servings: 4

Ingredients:

For the Salad:

- 4 large ripe tomatoes, sliced

- 8 ounces fresh mozzarella cheese, sliced

- 1/2 cup fresh basil leaves

- Salt and freshly ground black pepper to taste

For the Balsamic Glaze:

- 1/2 cup balsamic vinegar

- 2 tablespoons honey

Instructions:

1. Arrange the sliced tomatoes and fresh mozzarella cheese alternately on a serving platter.

2. If you're following a gastroparesis diet, make sure the tomatoes and mozzarella cheese are sliced into small, easily digestible pieces.

3. Tuck fresh basil leaves between the tomato and mozzarella slices.

4. Sprinkle the salad with a pinch of salt and freshly ground black pepper to taste.

5. In a small saucepan, prepare the balsamic glaze. Add 1/2 cup of balsamic vinegar and two tablespoons of honey.

6. If you're following a gastroparesis diet, make sure the balsamic glaze is smooth and free of any lumps.

7. Heat the mixture over low heat, stirring continuously until it thickens and reduces by half, which should take about 5-7 minutes.

8. Take out the balsamic glaze from the heat and let it cool slightly.

9. Drizzle the balsamic glaze over the Caprese salad.

10. Serve the Caprese Salad with Balsamic Glaze immediately while the glaze is still warm or at a temperature suitable for your diet.

Nutritional Information (per serving):

- Carbohydrates: 20g

- Fats: 20g

- Fiber: 2g

- Sodium: 340mg

- Protein: 12g

Jicama and Cucumber Salad

Prep Time: 15 minutes
Cook Time: 0 minutes
Number of Servings: 4

Ingredients:

For the Salad:

- 2 cups jicama, peeled and julienned

- 2 cups cucumber, peeled, seeded, and julienned

- 1/2 cup red bell pepper, thinly sliced

- 1/4 cup fresh cilantro leaves, chopped

For the Dressing:

- 2 tablespoons fresh lime juice

- 2 tablespoons extra-virgin olive oil

- 1 teaspoon honey

- 1/2 teaspoon ground cumin

- A pinch of salt and pepper

Instructions:

1. In a large bowl, add the julienned jicama, julienned cucumber, thinly sliced red bell pepper, and chopped fresh cilantro leaves.

2. If you're following a gastroparesis diet, ensure that the jicama, cucumber, and red bell pepper are finely julienned to aid in digestion.

3. In a separate small bowl, prepare the dressing. Whisk two tablespoons of fresh lime juice, two tablespoons of extra-virgin olive oil, one teaspoon of honey, 1/2 teaspoon of ground cumin, and a pinch of salt and pepper until well combined.

4. Pour the dressing over the salad mixture.

5. Gently toss the salad to ensure all ingredients are coated with the dressing.

6. Serve the Jicama and Cucumber Salad immediately at a temperature suitable for your diet.

Nutritional Information (per serving):

- Carbohydrates: 16g

- Fats: 7g

- Fiber: 8g

- Sodium: 50mg

- Protein: 1g

Thai-Inspired Cabbage Salad

Prep Time: 15 minutes
Cook Time: 0 minutes
Number of Servings: 4

Ingredients:

For the Salad:

- 4 cups shredded green cabbage

- 1 cup shredded carrots

- 1/2 cup thinly sliced red bell pepper

- 1/4 cup chopped fresh cilantro

- 1/4 cup chopped fresh mint

- 1/4 cup chopped roasted peanuts (optional, omit if needed)

For the Dressing:

- 3 tablespoons fresh lime juice

- 2 tablespoons fish sauce (or soy sauce for a vegetarian option)

- 1 tablespoon honey

- 1 teaspoon grated fresh ginger

- 1 small red chili pepper, finely chopped (adjust to taste)

- A pinch of salt

Instructions:

1. In a large bowl, add the shredded green cabbage, shredded carrots, thinly sliced red bell pepper, chopped fresh cilantro, and chopped fresh mint.

2. If you're following a gastroparesis diet, ensure that the cabbage, carrots, and red bell pepper are finely shredded to aid in digestion.

3. In a separate small bowl, prepare the dressing. Whisk three tablespoons of fresh lime juice, two tablespoons of fish sauce (or soy sauce for a vegetarian option), one tablespoon of honey, one teaspoon of grated fresh ginger, the finely chopped small red chili pepper (adjust the amount to your spice preference), and a pinch of salt until well combined.

4. Pour the dressing over the salad mixture.

5. Gently toss the salad to ensure all ingredients are coated with the dressing.

6. If using, sprinkle the chopped roasted peanuts over the salad. (Note: Skip this step if nuts are not suitable for your gastroparesis diet.)

7. Serve the Thai-Inspired Cabbage Salad immediately at a temperature suitable for your diet.

Nutritional Information (per serving):

- Carbohydrates: 17g

- Fats: 5g

- Fiber: 4g

- Sodium: 893mg (adjust by reducing fish sauce/soy sauce for lower sodium content)

- Protein: 4g

Mixed Greens with Raspberry Walnut Vinaigrette
Prep Time: 10 minutes
Cook Time: 0 minutes
Number of Servings: 4

Ingredients:

For the Salad:

- 8 cups mixed salad greens (e.g., lettuce, spinach, arugula)

- 1/2 cup fresh raspberries

- 1/4 cup crumbled goat cheese (optional, omit if needed)

- 1/4 cup chopped walnuts (optional, omit if needed)

For the Raspberry Walnut Vinaigrette:

- 1/2 cup fresh raspberries

- 3 tablespoons extra-virgin olive oil

- 2 tablespoons red wine vinegar

- 1 tablespoon honey

- A pinch of salt and freshly ground black pepper

Instructions:

1. In a large salad bowl, place the mixed salad greens.

2. If you're following a gastroparesis diet, make sure the salad greens are well-washed and free of tough stems.

3. Add the fresh raspberries to the salad greens.

4. If using, sprinkle the crumbled goat cheese over the salad. (Note: Skip this step if dairy is not suitable for your gastroparesis diet.)

5. If using, scatter the chopped walnuts over the salad. (Note: Skip this step if nuts are not suitable for your gastroparesis diet.)

6. In a blender or food processor, add 1/2 cup of fresh raspberries, three tablespoons of extra-virgin olive oil, two tablespoons of red wine vinegar, one tablespoon of honey, a pinch of salt, and freshly ground black pepper to taste.

7. Blend until the vinaigrette is smooth and well combined.

8. Drizzle the Raspberry Walnut Vinaigrette over the salad.

9. Gently toss the salad to ensure all ingredients are coated with the dressing.

10. Serve the Mixed Greens with Raspberry Walnut Vinaigrette immediately at a temperature suitable for your diet.

Nutritional Information (per serving):

- Carbohydrates: 13g

- Fats: 16g

- Fiber: 3g

- Sodium: 105mg

- Protein: 3g

Mixed Greens with Grilled Chicken and Raspberry Vinaigrette

Prep Time: 15 minutes
Cook Time: 15 minutes
Number of Servings: 4

Ingredients:

For the Salad:

- 8 cups mixed salad greens (e.g., lettuce, spinach, arugula)
- 2 boneless, skinless chicken breasts
- 1 tablespoon olive oil
- Salt and freshly ground black pepper to taste

For the Raspberry Vinaigrette:

- 1/2 cup fresh raspberries
- 3 tablespoons extra-virgin olive oil
- 2 tablespoons red wine vinegar
- 1 tablespoon honey
- A pinch of salt and freshly ground black pepper

Instructions:

1. Preheat your grill to medium-high heat.
2. Season the boneless, skinless chicken breasts with salt and freshly ground black pepper to taste.
3. Grill the chicken breasts for about 6-7 minutes per side, or until properly cooked and no longer pink in the center. The internal temperature should reach 165°F (74°C).
4. While the chicken is grilling, in a blender or food processor, add 1/2 cup of fresh raspberries, three tablespoons of extra-virgin olive oil, two tablespoons of red wine vinegar, one tablespoon of honey, a pinch of salt, and freshly ground black pepper to taste.
5. Blend until the vinaigrette is smooth and well combined.
6. In a large salad bowl, place the mixed salad greens.
7. If you're following a gastroparesis diet, make sure the salad greens are well-washed and free of tough stems.
8. Once the chicken is cooked, remove it from the grill and let it rest for a few minutes. Then, slice it into thin strips.

9. Add the sliced grilled chicken to the salad greens.

10. Drizzle the Raspberry Vinaigrette over the salad.

11. Gently toss the salad to ensure all ingredients are coated with the dressing.

12. Serve the Mixed Greens with Grilled Chicken and Raspberry Vinaigrette immediately at a temperature suitable for your diet.

Nutritional Information (per serving):

- Carbohydrates: 11g

- Fats: 20g

- Fiber: 2g

- Sodium: 110mg

- Protein: 24g

Avocado and Grapefruit Salad

Prep Time: 15 minutes
Cook Time: 0 minutes
Number of Servings: 4

Ingredients:

For the Salad:

- 2 ripe avocados, diced

- 2 grapefruits, segmented and membranes removed

- 4 cups mixed salad greens (e.g., lettuce, spinach, arugula)

- 1/4 cup thinly sliced red onion

- 1/4 cup chopped fresh cilantro

- 1/4 cup chopped unsalted pistachios (optional, omit if needed)

For the Dressing:

- 2 tablespoons extra-virgin olive oil

- 2 tablespoons fresh grapefruit juice

- 1 teaspoon honey

- A pinch of salt and freshly ground black pepper

Instructions:

1. In a large salad bowl, place the mixed salad greens.

2. If you're following a gastroparesis diet, make sure the salad greens are well-washed and free of tough stems.

3. Dice the ripe avocados and add them to the salad greens.

4. Segment the grapefruits and take out the membranes. Add the grapefruit segments to the salad.

5. Thinly slice the red onion and sprinkle it over the salad.

6. If using, sprinkle the chopped unsalted pistachios over the salad. (Note: Skip this step if nuts are not suitable for your gastroparesis diet.)

7. In a small bowl, prepare the dressing by whisking together two tablespoons of extra-virgin olive oil, two tablespoons of fresh grapefruit juice, one teaspoon of honey, a pinch of salt, and freshly ground black pepper to taste.

8. Drizzle the dressing over the salad.

9. Gently toss the salad to ensure all ingredients are coated with the dressing.

10. Serve the Avocado and Grapefruit Salad immediately at a temperature suitable for your diet.

Nutritional Information (per serving):

- Carbohydrates: 24g

- Fats: 16g

- Fiber: 8g

- Sodium: 170mg

- Protein: 4g

Quinoa and Roasted Vegetable Salad

Prep Time: 15 minutes
Cook Time: 25 minutes
Number of Servings: 4

Ingredients:

For the Salad:

- 1 cup quinoa
- 2 cups water or vegetable broth
- 2 cups mixed roasted vegetables (e.g., bell peppers, zucchini, carrots)
- 1/2 cup chopped fresh spinach
- 1/4 cup crumbled feta cheese (optional, omit if needed)
- 2 tablespoons chopped fresh basil
- 2 tablespoons chopped fresh parsley
- 2 tablespoons chopped fresh mint
- Salt and freshly ground black pepper to taste

For the Dressing:

- 3 tablespoons extra-virgin olive oil
- 2 tablespoons lemon juice
- 1 clove garlic, minced
- A pinch of salt and freshly ground black pepper

Instructions:

1. Rinse the quinoa under cold water in a fine-mesh strainer. Drain well.

2. In a medium saucepan, add the rinsed quinoa and two cups of water or vegetable broth. Bring to a boil over high heat.

3. Once boiling, reduce the heat to low, cover, and simmer for about 15-20 minutes, or until the quinoa is tender and has absorbed all the liquid.

4. While the quinoa is cooking, prepare the roasted vegetables. You can roast them in the oven at 400°F (200°C) for about 15-20 minutes, tossing them with a little olive oil, salt, and pepper, until tender and slightly caramelized. Alternatively, you can use leftover roasted vegetables.

5. In a large salad bowl, add the cooked quinoa, mixed roasted vegetables, chopped fresh spinach, crumbled feta cheese (if using), chopped fresh basil, chopped fresh parsley, and chopped fresh mint.

6. If you're following a gastroparesis diet, ensure that the roasted vegetables are finely chopped to aid in digestion.

7. In a small bowl, prepare the dressing by whisking together three tablespoons of extra-virgin olive oil, two tablespoons of lemon juice, minced garlic, a pinch of salt, and freshly ground black pepper to taste.

8. Drizzle the dressing over the salad.

9. Gently toss the salad to ensure all ingredients are coated with the dressing.

10. Serve the Quinoa and Roasted Vegetable Salad immediately at a temperature suitable for your diet.

Nutritional Information (per serving):

- Carbohydrates: 36g

- Fats: 14g

- Fiber: 6g

- Sodium: 260mg

- Protein: 8g

Cucumber and Mint Salad

Prep Time: 10 minutes
Cook Time: 0 minutes
Number of Servings: 4

Ingredients:

For the Salad:

- 4 cups thinly sliced cucumbers
- 1/4 cup thinly sliced red onion
- 1/4 cup chopped fresh mint leaves
- A pinch of salt

For the Dressing:

- 2 tablespoons fresh lime juice
- 2 tablespoons extra-virgin olive oil
- 1 teaspoon honey (optional, omit if needed)

Instructions:

1. In a large bowl, place the thinly sliced cucumbers.
2. If you're following a gastroparesis diet, ensure the cucumbers are thinly sliced and free of tough skin.
3. Add the thinly sliced red onion to the cucumbers.
4. In a separate small bowl, prepare the dressing by whisking together two tablespoons of fresh lime juice, two tablespoons of extra-virgin olive oil, and one teaspoon of honey (omit honey if not suitable for your diet).
5. If you're following a gastroparesis diet, make sure the dressing is smooth and free of any lumps.
6. Pour the dressing over the cucumber and red onion mixture.
7. Add the chopped fresh mint leaves to the salad.
8. Sprinkle a pinch of salt over the salad.
9. Gently toss the salad to ensure all ingredients are coated with the dressing.
10. Serve the Cucumber and Mint Salad immediately at a temperature suitable for your diet.

Nutritional Information (per serving):

- Carbohydrates: 5g

- Fats: 7g

- Fiber: 1g

- Sodium: 65mg

- Protein: 1g

Tuna Salad with Greek Yogurt Dressing

Prep Time: 15 minutes
Cook Time: 0 minutes
Number of Servings: 2

Ingredients:

For the Salad:

- 2 cans (5 ounces each) of canned tuna, drained

- 2 cups mixed salad greens (e.g., lettuce, spinach, arugula)

- 1/2 cucumber, diced

- 1/2 red bell pepper, diced

- 1/4 cup sliced black olives (optional, omit if needed)

- 1/4 cup chopped fresh parsley

- A pinch of salt and freshly ground black pepper

For the Greek Yogurt Dressing:

- 1/2 cup plain Greek yogurt

- 2 tablespoons lemon juice

- 1 tablespoon extra-virgin olive oil

- 1 clove garlic, minced

- 1/2 teaspoon dried dill (or one teaspoon fresh dill)

- A pinch of salt and freshly ground black pepper

Instructions:

1. In a large bowl, place the drained canned tuna.

2. If you're following a gastroparesis diet, ensure that the canned tuna is well-drained, and you can break it into smaller, easily digestible pieces if necessary.

3. Add the mixed salad greens to the bowl with the tuna.

4. Dice the cucumber and red bell pepper, and add them to the bowl.

5. If using, add the sliced black olives to the salad. (Note: Skip this step if olives are not suitable for your gastroparesis diet.)

6. Sprinkle the chopped fresh parsley over the salad.

7. Season the salad with a pinch of salt and freshly ground black pepper to taste.

8. In a separate small bowl, prepare the Greek Yogurt Dressing by whisking together 1/2 cup of plain Greek yogurt, two tablespoons of lemon juice, one tablespoon of extra-virgin olive oil, minced garlic, dried dill (or fresh dill), and a pinch of salt and freshly ground black pepper to taste.

9. If you're following a gastroparesis diet, ensure that the dressing is smooth and free of any lumps.

10. Drizzle the Greek Yogurt Dressing over the salad.

11. Gently toss the salad to ensure all ingredients are coated with the dressing.

12. Serve the Tuna Salad with Greek Yogurt Dressing immediately at a temperature suitable for your diet.

Nutritional Information (per serving):

- Carbohydrates: 11g

- Fats: 10g

- Fiber: 3g

- Sodium: 450mg

- Protein: 32g

Beet and Orange Salad

Prep Time: 15 minutes
Cook Time: 0 minutes
Number of Servings: 4

Ingredients:

For the Salad:

- 4 medium beets, cooked, peeled, and diced
- 2 large oranges, peeled, segmented, and membranes removed
- 4 cups mixed salad greens (e.g., lettuce, spinach, arugula)
- 1/4 cup thinly sliced red onion
- 1/4 cup chopped fresh parsley
- A pinch of salt and freshly ground black pepper

For the Dressing:

- 2 tablespoons extra-virgin olive oil
- 2 tablespoons red wine vinegar
- 1 teaspoon honey (optional, omit if needed)
- A pinch of salt and freshly ground black pepper

Instructions:

1. Begin by cooking the beets. You can either roast them in the oven or boil them until tender. Once cooked, peel the beets and dice them into small pieces.

2. If you're following a gastroparesis diet, ensure that the beets are cooked until very tender and diced into small, easily digestible pieces.

3. In a large bowl, place the diced beets.

4. Add the peeled and segmented oranges to the bowl with the beets. Make sure to remove any membranes from the oranges.

5. If you're following a gastroparesis diet, ensure that the orange segments are free of any tough membranes.

6. Add the mixed salad greens to the bowl.

7. Thinly slice the red onion and sprinkle it over the salad.

8. Sprinkle the chopped fresh parsley over the salad.

9. Season the salad with a pinch of salt and freshly ground black pepper to taste.

10. In a separate small bowl, prepare the dressing by whisking together two tablespoons of extra-virgin olive oil, two tablespoons of red wine vinegar, and one teaspoon of honey (omit honey if not suitable for your diet). Add a pinch of salt and freshly ground black pepper to taste.

11. Drizzle the dressing over the salad.

12. Gently toss the salad to ensure all ingredients are coated with the dressing.

13. Serve the Beet and Orange Salad immediately at a temperature suitable for your diet.

Nutritional Information (per serving):

- Carbohydrates: 27g

- Fats: 7g

- Fiber: 5g

- Sodium: 240mg

- Protein: 3g

Spinach and Strawberry Salad

Prep Time: 15 minutes
Cook Time: 0 minutes
Number of Servings: 4

Ingredients:

For the Salad:

- 8 cups fresh spinach leaves

- 2 cups fresh strawberries, hulled and sliced

- 1/4 cup thinly sliced red onion

- 1/4 cup chopped pecans (optional, omit if needed)

For the Dressing:

- 3 tablespoons extra-virgin olive oil
- 2 tablespoons balsamic vinegar
- 1 teaspoon honey (optional, omit if needed)
- A pinch of salt and freshly ground black pepper

Instructions:

1. In a large salad bowl, place the fresh spinach leaves.

2. If you're following a gastroparesis diet, ensure that the spinach leaves are fresh and free of any tough stems.

3. Add the sliced fresh strawberries to the bowl with the spinach.

4. Thinly slice the red onion and sprinkle it over the salad.

5. If using, add the chopped pecans to the salad. (Note: Skip this step if nuts are not suitable for your gastroparesis diet.)

6. In a separate small bowl, prepare the dressing by whisking together three tablespoons of extra-virgin olive oil, two tablespoons of balsamic vinegar, and one teaspoon of honey (omit honey if not suitable for your diet). Add a pinch of salt and freshly ground black pepper to taste.

7. If you're following a gastroparesis diet, ensure that the dressing is smooth and free of any lumps.

8. Drizzle the dressing over the salad.

9. Gently toss the salad to ensure all ingredients are coated with the dressing.

10. Serve the Spinach and Strawberry Salad immediately at a temperature suitable for your diet.

Nutritional Information (per serving):

- Carbohydrates: 14g
- Fats: 10g
- Fiber: 4g

- Sodium: 120mg

- Protein: 3g

Watermelon and Feta Salad

Prep Time: 15 minutes
Cook Time: 0 minutes
Number of Servings: 4

Ingredients:

For the Salad:

- 4 cups diced seedless watermelon

- 1 cup crumbled feta cheese

- 1/4 cup fresh mint leaves, chopped

- 1/4 cup thinly sliced red onion

- A pinch of salt and freshly ground black pepper

For the Dressing:

- 2 tablespoons extra-virgin olive oil

- 2 tablespoons balsamic vinegar

- A pinch of salt and freshly ground black pepper

Instructions:

1. In a large bowl, place the diced seedless watermelon.

2. If you're following a gastroparesis diet, ensure that the watermelon is diced into small, easily digestible pieces.

3. Add the crumbled feta cheese to the bowl with the watermelon.

4. Sprinkle the chopped fresh mint leaves over the salad.

5. Thinly slice the red onion and sprinkle it over the salad.

6. Season the salad with a pinch of salt and freshly ground black pepper to taste.

7. In a separate small bowl, prepare the dressing by whisking together two tablespoons of extra-virgin olive oil and two tablespoons of balsamic vinegar. Add a pinch of salt and freshly ground black pepper to taste.

8. If you're following a gastroparesis diet, ensure that the dressing is smooth and free of any lumps.

9. Drizzle the dressing over the Watermelon and Feta Salad.

10. Gently toss the salad to ensure all ingredients are coated with the dressing.

11. Serve the Watermelon and Feta Salad immediately at a temperature suitable for your diet.

Nutritional Information (per serving):

- Carbohydrates: 18g

- Fats: 12g

- Fiber: 1g

- Sodium: 430mg

- Protein: 8g

MAIN COURSES

Lemon Dill Baked Cod

Prep Time: 15 minutes
Cook Time: 20 minutes
Servings: 4

Ingredients:

- 4 cod fillets (about 1 pound each)
- 2 tablespoons olive oil
- 2 lemons, juiced and zested
- 2 cloves garlic, minced
- 1 tablespoon fresh dill, chopped
- 1/2 teaspoon salt
- 1/4 teaspoon black pepper

Instructions:

1. Turn on your oven and set it to 375°F (190°C) and grease a baking dish with a small amount of olive oil.

2. Place the cod fillets in the prepared baking dish.

3. In a small bowl, whisk the olive oil, lemon juice, lemon zest, minced garlic, fresh dill, salt, and black pepper.

4. Pour the lemon dill mixture evenly over the cod fillets.

5. Cover the baking dish with aluminum foil.

6. Bake in the preheated oven for 15-20 minutes or until the cod flakes easily with a fork and reaches an internal temperature of 145°F (63°C).

7. Once cooked, take out the foil and broil the cod for an extra 2-3 minutes until the top is lightly browned.

8. Serve the lemon dill baked cod hot, garnished with extra fresh dill and lemon slices if desired.

Nutritional Information (per serving):

- Carbs: 2 grams
- Fats: 10 grams
- Fiber: 0 grams
- Sodium: 330 milligrams
- Protein: 25 grams

Turkey and Quinoa Stuffed Bell Peppers

Prep Time: 20 minutes
Cook Time: 45 minutes
Servings: 4

Ingredients:

- 4 large bell peppers, any color
- 1 cup quinoa, rinsed and drained
- 1 pound ground turkey
- 1 small onion, finely chopped
- 2 cloves garlic, minced
- 1 can (14.5 ounces) diced tomatoes, drained
- 1 cup low-sodium chicken broth
- 1 teaspoon dried oregano
- 1/2 teaspoon dried basil
- 1/2 teaspoon salt
- 1/4 teaspoon black pepper
- 1 cup shredded low-fat cheddar cheese (optional)

Instructions:

1. Turn on your oven and set it to 350°F (175°C).
2. Cut the tops off the bell peppers and take out the seeds and membranes. Set aside.

3. In a medium saucepan, add the quinoa and two cups of water. Bring to a boil, then reduce the heat to low, cover, and simmer for 15 minutes or until the quinoa is cooked and the water is absorbed. Take it out from heat and fluff with a fork.

4. In a large skillet, cook the ground turkey over medium-high heat until it's no longer pink. Break it into small pieces as it cooks. Drain any excess fat.

5. Add the finely chopped onion and minced garlic to the skillet with the turkey. Cook for about 3-4 minutes until the onion is translucent.

6. Stir in the drained diced tomatoes, cooked quinoa, dried oregano, dried basil, salt, and black pepper. Cook for an extra 2-3 minutes to allow the flavors to meld.

7. Pour the low-sodium chicken broth into the skillet mixture and stir until well combined. Simmer for 5-7 minutes or until most of the liquid is absorbed.

8. Stuff each of the bell peppers with the turkey and quinoa mixture.

9. Place the stuffed peppers in a baking dish and cover with aluminum foil.

10. Bake in the preheated oven for 30-35 minutes or until the peppers are tender.

11. If desired, take out the foil, sprinkle the shredded low-fat cheddar cheese on top of each pepper, and bake for an extra 5 minutes or until the cheese is melted and bubbly.

12. Serve the turkey and quinoa stuffed bell peppers hot.

Nutritional Information (per serving):

- Carbs: 33 grams
- Fats: 7 grams
- Fiber: 6 grams
- Sodium: 620 milligrams
- Protein: 30 grams

Creamy Chicken and Rice Casserole

Prep Time: 15 minutes
Cook Time: 45 minutes
Servings: 6

Ingredients:

- 1.5 pounds boneless, skinless chicken breasts, diced
- 1 cup long-grain white rice
- 2 cups low-sodium chicken broth
- 1 cup water
- 1 cup frozen peas
- 1 cup sliced carrots
- 1/2 cup diced celery
- 1/2 cup diced onion
- 2 cloves garlic, minced
- 1 cup low-fat Greek yogurt
- 1/2 cup grated Parmesan cheese
- 1/4 cup fresh parsley, chopped
- 1 teaspoon dried thyme
- 1/2 teaspoon salt
- 1/4 teaspoon black pepper
- 1/4 teaspoon paprika

Instructions:

1. Turn on your oven and set it to 375°F (190°C).

2. In a large skillet, heat a small amount of oil over medium-high heat. Add the diced chicken and cook until it's no longer pink, about 5-7 minutes. Take out the chicken from the skillet and set it aside.

3. In the same skillet, add the diced onion, minced garlic, sliced carrots, and diced celery. Sauté for about 5 minutes, or until the vegetables are slightly softened.

4. Add the white rice to the skillet and cook for an extra 2 minutes, stirring frequently.

5. Stir in the low-sodium chicken broth, water, frozen peas, dried thyme, salt, black pepper, and paprika. Bring the mixture to a simmer.

6. Return the cooked chicken to the skillet and mix everything together.

7. Transfer the mixture to a greased 9x13-inch baking dish.

8. In a separate bowl, add the low-fat Greek yogurt and grated Parmesan cheese. Spread this mixture evenly over the chicken and rice in the baking dish.

9. Cover the baking dish with aluminum foil.

10. Bake in the preheated oven for 30 minutes.

11. Take out the foil and continue to bake for an extra 10-15 minutes, or until the top is golden and bubbly, and the rice is fully cooked.

12. Garnish the creamy chicken and rice casserole with fresh parsley before serving.

Nutritional Information (per serving):

- Carbs: 36 grams

- Fats: 8 grams

- Fiber: 3 grams

- Sodium: 490 milligrams

- Protein: 35 grams

Zucchini and Carrot Noodles with Pesto

Prep Time: 15 minutes
Cook Time: 10 minutes
Servings: 4

Ingredients:

- 2 large zucchinis
- 2 large carrots
- 1/2 cup fresh basil leaves
- 1/4 cup grated Parmesan cheese
- 1/4 cup pine nuts
- 2 cloves garlic, minced
- 1/4 cup olive oil
- 1/2 teaspoon salt
- 1/4 teaspoon black pepper
- 1/4 teaspoon red pepper flakes (optional)

Instructions:

1. Start by making the pesto sauce. In a food processor, add the fresh basil leaves, grated Parmesan cheese, pine nuts, minced garlic, olive oil, salt, and black pepper. Blend until you have a smooth pesto sauce. If desired, add the red pepper flakes for a hint of heat. Set the pesto aside.

2. Trim the ends of the zucchinis and carrots. Use a spiralizer or a vegetable peeler to create zucchini and carrot noodles. Set aside.

3. In a large skillet, heat a small amount of olive oil over medium heat.

4. Add the zucchini and carrot noodles to the skillet. Sauté for about 4-5 minutes, or until slightly softened but still have a bit of crunch.

5. Pour the prepared pesto sauce over the zucchini and carrot noodles. Toss everything together until the noodles are coated evenly with the pesto sauce.

6. Cook for an extra 2-3 minutes, allowing the noodles to absorb the flavors of the pesto.

7. Taste and adjust the seasoning with additional salt and black pepper if needed.

8. Serve the zucchini and carrot noodles with pesto hot, garnished with extra grated Parmesan cheese and pine nuts if desired.

Nutritional Information (per serving):

- Carbs: 10 grams

- Fats: 21 grams

- Fiber: 3 grams

- Sodium: 360 milligrams

- Protein: 6 grams

Ginger Teriyaki Tofu

Prep Time: 20 minutes
Cook Time: 20 minutes
Servings: 4

Ingredients:

- 1 block (14 ounces) extra-firm tofu

- 1/4 cup low-sodium soy sauce

- 2 tablespoons honey

- 1 tablespoon rice vinegar

- 1 teaspoon fresh ginger, grated

- 1 clove garlic, minced

- 1 tablespoon cornstarch

- 2 tablespoons water

- 2 tablespoons sesame oil

- 1/2 cup sliced green onions

- 1 tablespoon sesame seeds

- Cooked white rice for serving

Instructions:

1. Start by preparing the tofu. Drain the tofu block and wrap it in a clean kitchen towel. Place a heavy object, like a skillet or a can, on top of the tofu to press out excess liquid. Leave it for about 15 minutes.

2. While the tofu is pressing, prepare the teriyaki sauce. In a small bowl, whisk the low-sodium soy sauce, honey, rice vinegar, grated fresh ginger, and minced garlic.

3. In another small bowl, mix the cornstarch and water to create a slurry. Set both the sauce and the cornstarch slurry aside.

4. After pressing, cut the tofu into 1/2-inch cubes.

5. Heat the sesame oil in a large skillet or wok over medium-high heat.

6. Add the tofu cubes to the hot skillet and cook for about 4-5 minutes, or until golden brown on all sides.

7. Pour the prepared teriyaki sauce over the tofu cubes. Stir gently to coat the tofu evenly.

8. Allow the sauce to simmer for 2-3 minutes, thickening as it cooks.

9. Add the sliced green onions and sesame seeds to the skillet, reserving some for garnish.

10. Keep on cooking for an extra 1-2 minutes, until the green onions are slightly wilted.

11. Serve the ginger teriyaki tofu over cooked white rice, garnished with extra sliced green onions and sesame seeds.

Nutritional Information (per serving):

- Carbs: 20 grams

- Fats: 10 grams

- Fiber: 1 gram

- Sodium: 420 milligrams

- Protein: 9 grams

Baked Eggplant Parmesan (Gluten-Free)

Prep Time: 30 minutes
Cook Time: 30 minutes
Servings: 4

Ingredients:

- 1 large eggplant

- 1 cup gluten-free breadcrumbs

- 1/2 cup grated Parmesan cheese

- 1 teaspoon dried oregano

- 1 teaspoon dried basil

- 1/2 teaspoon garlic powder

- 1/2 teaspoon salt

- 1/4 teaspoon black pepper

- 2 large eggs

- 2 cups gluten-free marinara sauce

- 1 1/2 cups shredded mozzarella cheese

- Fresh basil leaves for garnish (optional)

Instructions:

1. Turn on your oven and set it to 375°F (190°C).

2. Slice the eggplant into 1/2-inch thick rounds.

3. In a shallow bowl, add the gluten-free breadcrumbs, grated Parmesan cheese, dried oregano, dried basil, garlic powder, salt, and black pepper. Mix sufficiently.

4. In another shallow bowl, beat the large eggs.

5. Dip each eggplant slice into the beaten eggs, allowing any excess to drip off.

6. Press each egg-coated eggplant slice into the breadcrumb mixture, ensuring both sides are well coated.

7. Place the breaded eggplant slices on a baking sheet lined with parchment paper.

8. Bake in the preheated oven for 20-25 minutes, flipping the slices halfway through, until golden and crispy.

9. In a separate saucepan, heat the gluten-free marinara sauce over low heat until warmed.

10. In a greased baking dish, spread a thin layer of marinara sauce.

11. Arrange the baked eggplant slices over the sauce in a single layer.

12. Pour the remaining marinara sauce evenly over the eggplant slices.

13. Sprinkle the shredded mozzarella cheese on top.

14. Bake for an extra 10-15 minutes, or until the cheese is melted and bubbly.

15. Garnish with fresh basil leaves if desired before serving.

Nutritional Information (per serving):

- Carbs: 29 grams

- Fats: 15 grams

- Fiber: 5 grams

- Sodium: 960 milligrams

- Protein: 19 grams

Spinach and Feta Stuffed Chicken Breast

Prep Time: 20 minutes
Cook Time: 30 minutes
Servings: 4

Ingredients:

- 4 boneless, skinless chicken breasts
- 2 cups fresh spinach leaves
- 1/2 cup crumbled feta cheese
- 1/4 cup diced sun-dried tomatoes (packed in oil, drained)
- 1 clove garlic, minced
- 1/2 teaspoon dried oregano
- 1/2 teaspoon dried basil
- 1/4 teaspoon salt
- 1/4 teaspoon black pepper
- 2 tablespoons olive oil

Instructions:

1. Turn on your oven and set it to 375°F (190°C).
2. In a large skillet, heat one tablespoon of olive oil over medium-high heat.
3. Add the minced garlic and cook for about 1 minute until fragrant.
4. Add the fresh spinach leaves to the skillet. Sauté for 2-3 minutes, or until the spinach is wilted. Take it out from heat.
5. In a mixing bowl, add the crumbled feta cheese, diced sun-dried tomatoes, dried oregano, dried basil, salt, and black pepper. Mix sufficiently.
6. Lay the chicken breasts flat on a cutting board. Slice a pocket horizontally through the thickest part of each chicken breast, being careful not to cut all the way through.
7. Stuff each chicken breast with an equal amount of the spinach and feta mixture.
8. Use toothpicks to secure the opening of each stuffed chicken breast.

9. In the same skillet you used for the spinach, heat the remaining one tablespoon of olive oil over medium-high heat.

10. Place the stuffed chicken breasts in the skillet and sear them for about 2-3 minutes on each side until golden brown.

11. Transfer the seared chicken breasts to a baking dish.

12. Bake in the preheated oven for 20-25 minutes or until the chicken reaches an internal temperature of 165°F (74°C) and is no longer pink in the center.

13. Take out the toothpicks before serving.

Nutritional Information (per serving):

- Carbs: 5 grams

- Fats: 16 grams

- Fiber: 1 gram

- Sodium: 420 milligrams

- Protein: 35 grams

Lentil and Butternut Squash Curry

Prep Time: 20 minutes
Cook Time: 30 minutes
Servings: 4

Ingredients:

- 1 cup dried green or brown lentils

- 2 cups diced butternut squash

- 1 tablespoon olive oil

- 1 medium onion, finely chopped

- 2 cloves garlic, minced

- 1-inch piece of fresh ginger, grated

- 2 tablespoons curry powder

- 1 teaspoon ground cumin

- 1/2 teaspoon ground coriander
- 1/4 teaspoon ground turmeric
- 1/4 teaspoon cayenne pepper (adjust to taste)
- 1 can (14.5 ounces) diced tomatoes
- 1 can (14 ounces) coconut milk
- Salt and black pepper to taste
- Fresh cilantro leaves for garnish (optional)

Instructions:

1. Rinse the dried lentils thoroughly and set them aside.
2. In a large pot, heat the olive oil over medium-high heat.
3. Add the finely chopped onion and sauté for about 3-4 minutes, until it becomes translucent.
4. Stir in the minced garlic and grated ginger. Cook for an extra 1-2 minutes until fragrant.
5. Add the curry powder, ground cumin, ground coriander, ground turmeric, and cayenne pepper to the pot. Stir sufficiently to coat the onions, garlic, and ginger with the spices.
6. Add the diced butternut squash and keep on cooking for 3-4 minutes, allowing the squash to slightly soften.
7. Pour in the diced tomatoes (including their juice) and the rinsed lentils. Mix everything together.
8. Add the can of coconut milk to the pot and stir until well combined.
9. Bring the mixture to a boil, then reduce the heat to low, cover the pot, and simmer for 20-25 minutes, or until the lentils are tender and the butternut squash is properly cooked.
10. Season the curry with salt and black pepper to taste.
11. Serve the Lentil and Butternut Squash Curry hot, garnished with fresh cilantro leaves if desired.

Nutritional Information (per serving):

- Carbs: 52 grams

- Fats: 19 grams

- Fiber: 14 grams

- Sodium: 380 milligrams

- Protein: 14 grams

Baked Trout with Herbed Butter

Prep Time: 15 minutes **Cook Time:** 20 minutes **Number of Servings:** 4

Ingredients:

- 4 trout fillets (6 ounces each)

- 2 tablespoons unsalted butter, softened

- 2 cloves garlic, minced

- 1 tablespoon fresh parsley, chopped

- 1 tablespoon fresh dill, chopped

- 1 tablespoon fresh chives, chopped

- 1 lemon, zest and juice

- Salt and pepper to taste

- 1/4 cup low-sodium chicken broth

- 1/4 cup dry white wine

Instructions:

1. Turn on your oven and set it to 375°F (190°C) and grease a baking dish.

2. In a small mixing bowl, add the softened unsalted butter, minced garlic, chopped fresh parsley, fresh dill, fresh chives, lemon zest, and juice. Mix sufficiently until all the ingredients are thoroughly incorporated.

3. Season the trout fillets with salt and pepper on both sides.

4. Place the seasoned trout fillets in the greased baking dish.

5. Spread the herbed butter mixture evenly over the top of each trout fillet.

6. Pour the low-sodium chicken broth and dry white wine into the bottom of the baking dish.

7. Cover the baking dish with aluminum foil, sealing it tightly.

8. Bake in the preheated oven for approximately 15-20 minutes, or until the trout flakes easily with a fork.

9. Take out the foil and broil for an extra 2-3 minutes, or until the herbed butter on top of the trout is slightly browned.

10. Serve the baked trout hot, drizzling some of the pan juices over each fillet.

Nutritional Information (Per Serving):

- Carbs: 2 grams

- Fats: 10 grams

- Fiber: 0 grams

- Sodium: 160 milligrams

- Protein: 33 grams

Shrimp Scampi with Zoodles

Prep Time: 15 minutes **Cook Time:** 10 minutes **Number of Servings:** 4

Ingredients:

- 1 pound large shrimp, peeled and deveined

- 4 medium zucchinis, spiralized into zoodles

- 4 cloves garlic, minced

- 3 tablespoons unsalted butter

- 3 tablespoons olive oil

- 1/4 cup dry white wine

- 1/4 cup fresh parsley, chopped

- 1 lemon, zest and juice

- Salt and pepper to taste

- Red pepper flakes (optional, for added heat)

Instructions:

1. In a large skillet, heat the olive oil and two tablespoons of unsalted butter over medium-high heat.

2. Add the minced garlic and sauté for about 1 minute, or until fragrant.

3. Add the shrimp to the skillet and cook for 2-3 minutes per side, or until they turn pink and opaque. Take out the shrimp from the skillet and set them aside.

4. In the same skillet, add the remaining tablespoon of unsalted butter. Once melted, add the spiralized zucchini (zoodles) and sauté for 2-3 minutes until they begin to soften.

5. Pour in the dry white wine, lemon zest, and lemon juice. Stir and cook for an extra 2 minutes, allowing the flavors to meld and the zoodles to absorb some of the liquid.

6. Return the cooked shrimp to the skillet and stir to combine. Cook for an extra 1-2 minutes to heat the shrimp through.

7. Season with salt, pepper, and red pepper flakes (if desired) to taste.

8. Sprinkle the chopped fresh parsley over the top and give it a final stir.

9. Serve the Shrimp Scampi over the zoodles, ensuring to distribute the sauce evenly.

Nutritional Information (Per Serving):

- Carbs: 10 grams

- Fats: 16 grams

- Fiber: 2 grams

- Sodium: 232 milligrams

- Protein: 23 grams

Baked Salmon with Lemon-Dill Sauce

Prep Time: 10 minutes **Cook Time:** 15 minutes **Number of Servings:** 4

Ingredients:

- 4 salmon fillets (6 ounces each)

- 1 lemon, sliced

- Salt and pepper to taste

- For the Lemon-Dill Sauce:

    - 1/2 cup plain Greek yogurt

    - 1 tablespoon fresh dill, finely chopped

    - 1 teaspoon lemon zest

    - 2 tablespoons lemon juice

    - 1 clove garlic, minced

    - Salt and pepper to taste

Instructions:

1. Turn on your oven and set it to 375°F (190°C) and line a baking sheet with parchment paper.

2. Season the salmon fillets with salt and pepper on both sides.

3. Place the salmon fillets on the prepared baking sheet.

4. Lay lemon slices on top of each salmon fillet.

5. In a small bowl, add the plain Greek yogurt, finely chopped fresh dill, lemon zest, lemon juice, minced garlic, salt, and pepper. Mix until well combined to make the Lemon-Dill Sauce.

6. Spoon the Lemon-Dill Sauce evenly over each salmon fillet, covering them.

7. Bake the salmon in the preheated oven for approximately 15 minutes, or until the salmon flakes easily with a fork and reaches an internal temperature of 145°F (63°C).

8. Once done, take out the salmon from the oven and let it rest for a minute.

9. Serve the Baked Salmon with Lemon-Dill Sauce hot, and you can drizzle extra sauce over the top if desired.

Nutritional Information (Per Serving):

- Carbs: 3 grams

- Fats: 12 grams

- Fiber: 0 grams

- Sodium: 215 milligrams

- Protein: 32 grams

Turkey and Rice Casserole

Prep Time: 15 minutes **Cook Time:** 45 minutes **Number of Servings:** 6

Ingredients:

- 1 pound ground turkey

- 1 cup white rice

- 2 cups low-sodium chicken broth

- 1 cup carrots, diced

- 1 cup peas

- 1 cup celery, diced

- 1/2 cup onion, finely chopped

- 2 cloves garlic, minced

- 1 teaspoon dried thyme

- 1 teaspoon dried rosemary

- Salt and pepper to taste

- 1 cup shredded cheddar cheese (optional, for topping)

Instructions:

1. Turn on your oven and set it to 350°F (175°C).

2. In a large skillet, cook the ground turkey over medium heat until it's no longer pink. Break it into crumbles as it cooks. Drain any excess fat if necessary.

3. In a separate saucepan, add the white rice and low-sodium chicken broth. Bring it to a boil, then reduce the heat to low, cover, and simmer for 15 minutes or until the rice is cooked and the liquid is absorbed.

4. In the same skillet where you cooked the turkey, add the diced carrots, peas, celery, chopped onion, and minced garlic. Sauté until the vegetables are tender, about 5 minutes.

5. Stir in the dried thyme, dried rosemary, salt, and pepper.

6. In a large mixing bowl, add the cooked ground turkey, cooked rice, and sautéed vegetable mixture. Mix everything together thoroughly.

7. Transfer the mixture to a greased 9x13-inch baking dish.

8. If desired, sprinkle the shredded cheddar cheese evenly over the top of the casserole.

9. Cover the baking dish with foil and bake in the preheated oven for 25-30 minutes, or until the casserole is heated through and the cheese is melted (if using).

10. Serve the Turkey and Rice Casserole hot, and portion it according to your dietary needs.

Nutritional Information (Per Serving):

- Carbs: 27 grams

- Fats: 9 grams

- Fiber: 3 grams

- Sodium: 231 milligrams

- Protein: 20 grams

Zucchini Noodles with Pesto

Prep Time: 15 minutes **Cook Time:** 10 minutes **Number of Servings:** 4

Ingredients:

- 4 medium zucchinis, spiralized into noodles (zoodles)
- 2 cups fresh basil leaves
- 1/2 cup grated Parmesan cheese
- 1/4 cup pine nuts
- 2 cloves garlic, minced
- 1/2 cup extra-virgin olive oil
- 1 tablespoon fresh lemon juice
- Salt and pepper to taste
- Grated Parmesan cheese for garnish (optional)

Instructions:

1. In a large skillet, heat a small amount of olive oil over medium-high heat.

2. Add the spiralized zucchini noodles (zoodles) to the skillet and sauté for about 2-3 minutes, or until they start to soften. Take them out from the skillet and set them aside.

3. In a food processor, add the fresh basil leaves, grated Parmesan cheese, pine nuts, minced garlic, and a pinch of salt and pepper.

4. Pulse the ingredients in the food processor while slowly drizzling in the extra-virgin olive oil. Continue to blend until you have a smooth pesto sauce.

5. Add fresh lemon juice to the pesto sauce and pulse again to combine.

6. Taste the pesto and adjust the seasoning with additional salt and pepper if needed.

7. Return the sautéed zucchini noodles (zoodles) to the skillet.

8. Pour the pesto sauce over the zoodles and toss to coat them evenly.

9. Cook for an extra 2-3 minutes, or until the zoodles are heated through.

10. Serve the Zucchini Noodles with Pesto hot, garnished with additional grated Parmesan cheese if desired.

Nutritional Information (Per Serving):

- Carbs: 7 grams

- Fats: 31 grams

- Fiber: 2 grams

- Sodium: 210 milligrams

- Protein: 6 grams

Baked Cod with Herbed Butter

Prep Time: 15 minutes **Cook Time:** 20 minutes **Number of Servings:** 4

Ingredients:

- 4 cod fillets (6 ounces each)

- 2 tablespoons unsalted butter, softened

- 2 cloves garlic, minced

- 1 tablespoon fresh parsley, chopped

- 1 tablespoon fresh dill, chopped

- 1 tablespoon fresh chives, chopped

- 1 lemon, zest and juice

- Salt and pepper to taste

- 1/4 cup low-sodium chicken broth

- 1/4 cup dry white wine

Instructions:

1. Turn on your oven and set it to 375°F (190°C) and grease a baking dish.

2. In a small mixing bowl, add the softened unsalted butter, minced garlic, chopped fresh parsley, fresh dill, fresh chives, lemon zest, and lemon juice. Mix sufficiently until all the ingredients are thoroughly incorporated.

3. Season the cod fillets with salt and pepper on both sides.

4. Place the seasoned cod fillets in the greased baking dish.

5. Spread the herbed butter mixture evenly over the top of each cod fillet.

6. Pour the low-sodium chicken broth and dry white wine into the bottom of the baking dish.

7. Cover the baking dish with aluminum foil, sealing it tightly.

8. Bake in the preheated oven for approximately 15-20 minutes, or until the cod flakes easily with a fork.

9. Take out the foil and broil for an extra 2-3 minutes, or until the herbed butter on top of the cod is slightly browned.

10. Serve the baked cod hot, drizzling some of the pan juices over each fillet.

Nutritional Information (Per Serving):

- Carbs: 2 grams

- Fats: 10 grams

- Fiber: 0 grams

- Sodium: 160 milligrams

- Protein: 33 grams

Quiche with a Gluten-Free Crust

Prep Time: 20 minutes **Cook Time:** 45 minutes **Number of Servings:** 6

Ingredients:

For the Crust:

- 1 1/2 cups gluten-free all-purpose flour

- 1/2 cup unsalted butter, cold and cubed
- 1/4 teaspoon salt
- 1/4 cup ice water

For the Filling:

- 4 large eggs
- 1 cup lactose-free milk
- 1 cup spinach, finely chopped
- 1/2 cup cooked bacon, diced
- 1/2 cup Swiss cheese, shredded
- 1/4 cup green onions, thinly sliced
- Salt and pepper to taste
- Pinch of nutmeg (optional)

Instructions:

Making the Gluten-Free Crust:

1. In a food processor, add the gluten-free all-purpose flour, cold and cubed unsalted butter, and salt. Pulse until the mixture resembles coarse crumbs.

2. While pulsing, gradually add the ice water until the dough begins to come together.

3. Turn the dough out onto a clean surface and gently knead it a few times to bring it together into a ball.

4. Flatten the dough into a disk, wrap it in plastic wrap, and refrigerate for at least 30 minutes.

5. Turn on your oven and set it to 375°F (190°C).

6. Roll out the chilled dough on a gluten-free floured surface to fit a 9-inch pie dish.

7. Carefully transfer the crust to the pie dish, press it into place, and trim any excess hanging over the edges.

Making the Filling:

8. In a mixing bowl, whisk the large eggs, lactose-free milk, and a pinch of nutmeg (if using). Season with salt and pepper to taste.

9. Sprinkle the finely chopped spinach, diced cooked bacon, shredded Swiss cheese, and thinly sliced green onions evenly over the crust.

10. Pour the egg mixture over the filling ingredients in the crust.

11. Bake in the preheated oven for 40-45 minutes, or until the quiche is set in the center and the top is lightly golden.

12. Allow the quiche to cool for a few minutes before slicing and serving.

Nutritional Information (Per Serving):

- Carbs: 29 grams

- Fats: 24 grams

- Fiber: 3 grams

- Sodium: 425 milligrams

- Protein: 16 grams

SIDE DISHES

Mashed Sweet Potatoes with Cinnamon

Prep Time: 15 minutes

Cook Time: 30 minutes

Servings: 4

Ingredients:

- 4 medium-sized sweet potatoes, peeled and diced
- 1/4 cup unsweetened almond milk
- 2 tablespoons olive oil
- 1/2 teaspoon ground cinnamon
- 1/4 teaspoon salt
- 1/8 teaspoon ground black pepper

Instructions:

1. Place the diced sweet potatoes in a large pot and cover them with water. Bring the water to a boil over high heat.

2. Reduce the heat to medium and let the sweet potatoes simmer for about 15-20 minutes, or until tender when pierced with a fork.

3. Drain the sweet potatoes thoroughly.

4. In a large mixing bowl, add the drained sweet potatoes, almond milk, olive oil, ground cinnamon, salt, and ground black pepper.

5. Use a potato masher or a fork to mash the sweet potatoes until they reach your desired consistency. For a smoother texture, you can use a hand mixer.

6. Taste the mashed sweet potatoes and adjust the seasoning if necessary, adding more cinnamon, salt, or pepper to taste.

7. Serve the mashed sweet potatoes with a sprinkle of additional cinnamon on top, if desired.

Nutritional Information (per serving):

- Carbs: 40g
- Fats: 7g
- Fiber: 6g
- Sodium: 165mg
- Protein: 2g

Roasted Brussels Sprouts with Pecans

Prep Time: 10 minutes

Cook Time: 25 minutes

Servings: 4

Ingredients:

- 1 pound Brussels sprouts, trimmed and halved
- 1/4 cup pecans, roughly chopped
- 2 tablespoons olive oil
- 1 tablespoon maple syrup
- 1/4 teaspoon salt
- 1/8 teaspoon ground black pepper

Instructions:

1. Preheat the oven to 400°F (200°C).

2. In a large mixing bowl, add the halved Brussels sprouts, chopped pecans, olive oil, maple syrup, salt, and ground black pepper. Toss well to coat the Brussels sprouts and pecans evenly.

3. Spread the Brussels sprouts and pecans in a single layer on a baking sheet.

4. Roast in the preheated oven for about 20-25 minutes or until the Brussels sprouts are tender and lightly browned, stirring halfway through.

5. Remove from the oven and let them cool slightly before serving.

Nutritional Information (per serving):

- Carbs: 15g
- Fats: 9g
- Fiber: 6g
- Sodium: 153mg
- Protein: 5g

Sautéed Green Beans with Almonds

Prep Time: 10 minutes

Cook Time: 15 minutes

Servings: 4

Ingredients:

- 1 pound fresh green beans, trimmed and halved
- 1/4 cup slivered almonds
- 2 tablespoons unsalted butter
- 1 clove garlic, minced
- 1/4 teaspoon salt
- 1/8 teaspoon ground black pepper

Instructions:

1. In a large skillet, melt the unsalted butter over medium heat.

2. Add the minced garlic to the skillet and sauté for about 1 minute until it becomes fragrant but not browned.

3. Add the trimmed and halved green beans to the skillet.

4. Sauté the green beans in the butter and garlic mixture for approximately 8-10 minutes, or until tender-crisp. Stir occasionally to ensure even cooking.

5. While the green beans are cooking, in a separate small pan, toast the slivered almonds over medium-low heat for 3-4 minutes, or until they turn lightly golden. Keep a close eye on them to prevent burning.

6. Once the green beans are cooked to your desired level of tenderness, season them with salt and ground black pepper. Toss to coat evenly.

7. Transfer the sautéed green beans to a serving dish and sprinkle the toasted slivered almonds over the top.

Nutritional Information (per serving):

- Carbs: 9g

- Fats: 9g

- Fiber: 4g

- Sodium: 154mg

- Protein: 3g

Lemon Herb Quinoa Salad

Prep Time: 15 minutes

Cook Time: 15 minutes

Servings: 4

Ingredients:

- 1 cup quinoa

- 2 cups water

- 1 lemon, zest and juice

- 2 tablespoons olive oil

- 1/4 cup fresh parsley, finely chopped

- 1/4 cup fresh mint, finely chopped

- 1/4 teaspoon salt

- 1/8 teaspoon ground black pepper

- 1/4 cup cucumber, finely diced
- 1/4 cup red bell pepper, finely diced
- 1/4 cup cherry tomatoes, quartered
- 1/4 cup crumbled feta cheese (optional)

Instructions:

1. Rinse the quinoa thoroughly under cold water using a fine-mesh sieve.

2. In a medium saucepan, bring two cups of water to a boil. Add the rinsed quinoa and reduce the heat to low. Cover and simmer for about 12-15 minutes, or until the quinoa is cooked and the water is absorbed.

3. While the quinoa is cooking, prepare the dressing. In a small bowl, whisk the lemon zest, lemon juice, olive oil, finely chopped parsley, finely chopped mint, salt, and ground black pepper. Set aside.

4. Once the quinoa is cooked, fluff it with a fork and let it cool to room temperature.

5. In a large mixing bowl, add the cooked quinoa, finely diced cucumber, finely diced red bell pepper, and quartered cherry tomatoes.

6. Pour the prepared lemon herb dressing over the quinoa and vegetables. Toss well to coat all the ingredients evenly.

7. If desired, sprinkle crumbled feta cheese on top of the salad.

8. Serve the Lemon Herb Quinoa Salad chilled or at room temperature.

Nutritional Information (per serving):

- Carbs: 34g
- Fats: 9g
- Fiber: 4g
- Sodium: 191mg

- Protein: 7g

Lemon Herb Quinoa Salad

Prep Time: 15 minutes

Cook Time: 15 minutes

Servings: 4

Ingredients:

- 1 cup quinoa
- 2 cups water
- Zest and juice of 1 lemon
- 2 tablespoons olive oil
- 1/4 cup fresh parsley, finely chopped
- 1/4 cup fresh mint, finely chopped
- 1/4 teaspoon salt
- 1/8 teaspoon ground black pepper
- 1/4 cup cucumber, finely diced
- 1/4 cup red bell pepper, finely diced
- 1/4 cup cherry tomatoes, quartered
- 1/4 cup crumbled feta cheese (optional)

Instructions:

1. Rinse the quinoa thoroughly under cold water using a fine-mesh sieve.

2. In a medium saucepan, bring two cups of water to a boil. Add the rinsed quinoa and reduce the heat to low. Cover and simmer for about 12-15 minutes, or until the quinoa is cooked and the water is absorbed.

3. While the quinoa is cooking, prepare the dressing. In a small bowl, whisk the lemon zest, lemon juice, olive oil, finely

chopped parsley, finely chopped mint, salt, and ground black pepper. Set aside.

4. Once the quinoa is cooked, fluff it with a fork and let it cool to room temperature.

5. In a large mixing bowl, add the cooked quinoa, finely diced cucumber, finely diced red bell pepper, and quartered cherry tomatoes.

6. Pour the prepared lemon herb dressing over the quinoa and vegetables. Toss well to coat all the ingredients evenly.

7. If desired, sprinkle crumbled feta cheese on top of the salad.

8. Serve the Lemon Herb Quinoa Salad chilled or at room temperature.

Nutritional Information (per serving):

- Carbohydrates: 34g
- Fats: 9g
- Fiber: 4g
- Sodium: 191mg
- Protein: 7g

Grilled Asparagus with Garlic Butter

Prep Time: 10 minutes

Cook Time: 10 minutes

Servings: 4

Ingredients:

- 1 pound fresh asparagus spears, trimmed
- 2 tablespoons unsalted butter
- 2 cloves garlic, minced
- 1/4 teaspoon salt
- 1/8 teaspoon ground black pepper

- 1 tablespoon olive oil
- Lemon wedges for garnish (optional)

Instructions:

1. Preheat the grill to medium-high heat.

2. In a small saucepan, melt the unsalted butter over low heat. Add the minced garlic and cook for about 1-2 minutes, or until the garlic is fragrant. Take it out from heat and set aside.

3. Place the trimmed asparagus spears in a large mixing bowl. Drizzle olive oil over the asparagus and toss them to coat evenly.

4. Season the asparagus with salt and ground black pepper.

5. Arrange the asparagus spears on the preheated grill. Grill for about 4-5 minutes on each side, or until tender and slightly charred.

6. During the last minute of grilling, brush the melted garlic butter over the asparagus, turning them to ensure even coating.

7. Take out the grilled asparagus from the grill and transfer them to a serving platter.

8. Garnish with lemon wedges, if desired.

Nutritional Information (per serving):

- Carbs: 6g
- Fats: 8g
- Fiber: 3g
- Sodium: 158mg
- Protein: 3g

Steamed Artichokes with Lemon Aioli

Prep Time: 15 minutes

Cook Time: 45 minutes

Servings: 2

Ingredients:

- 2 large artichokes
- 1 lemon, sliced
- 1/2 cup mayonnaise
- 1 clove garlic, minced
- 1 tablespoon fresh lemon juice
- 1/4 teaspoon salt
- 1/8 teaspoon ground black pepper

Instructions:

1. Start by preparing the artichokes. Trim off the top inch of each artichoke, then use kitchen scissors to trim the sharp tips from the leaves. Cut the stem off flush with the base so the artichokes can stand upright.

2. Place a steamer basket in a large pot filled with about 2 inches of water. Add the sliced lemon to the water.

3. Set the prepared artichokes in the steamer basket, standing upright.

4. Cover the pot with a lid and bring the water to a simmer over medium-high heat. Steam the artichokes for about 35-45 minutes or until a leaf near the center pulls out easily.

5. While the artichokes are steaming, prepare the lemon aioli. In a small bowl, add the mayonnaise, minced garlic, fresh lemon juice, salt, and ground black pepper. Mix sufficiently. Adjust the seasoning to taste.

6. Once the artichokes are tender, take them out from the steamer and let them cool slightly.

7. Serve the steamed artichokes warm with the lemon aioli for dipping. To eat, peel off the leaves one at a time and dip the base of each leaf into the aioli. When you reach the tender inner leaves, take them out all at once to reveal the heart. Scoop out the fuzzy choke, and the heart is ready to eat.

Nutritional Information (per serving):

- Carbs: 11g
- Fats: 43g
- Fiber: 7g
- Sodium: 542mg
- Protein: 2g

Mashed Turnips with Chives

Prep Time: 10 minutes

Cook Time: 20 minutes

Servings: 4

Ingredients:

- 4 medium-sized turnips, peeled and diced
- 2 tablespoons unsalted butter
- 2 tablespoons fresh chives, finely chopped
- 1/4 teaspoon salt
- 1/8 teaspoon ground black pepper

Instructions:

1. Begin by peeling the turnips and cutting them into evenly sized chunks.
2. Place the diced turnips in a large pot and cover them with water.
3. Bring the water to a boil over high heat, then reduce the heat to medium and let the turnips simmer for about 15-20 minutes, or until tender when pierced with a fork.
4. Drain the cooked turnips thoroughly.
5. In the same pot or a mixing bowl, add the drained turnips, unsalted butter, finely chopped chives, salt, and ground black pepper.

6. Use a potato masher or a fork to mash the turnips until they reach your desired consistency. You can leave some texture or make them smooth, depending on your preference.

7. Taste the mashed turnips and adjust the seasoning if needed, adding more salt and pepper to taste.

8. Serve the Mashed Turnips with Chives as a delicious and comforting side dish.

Nutritional Information (per serving):

- Carbs: 13g

- Fats: 5g

- Fiber: 4g

- Sodium: 191mg

- Protein: 1g

Creamy Corn Pudding

Prep Time: 15 minutes

Cook Time: 45 minutes

Servings: 6

Ingredients:

- 4 cups fresh or frozen corn kernels

- 3 large eggs

- 1/4 cup unsalted butter, melted

- 1 cup whole milk

- 1/4 cup cornmeal

- 1/4 cup granulated sugar

- 1/2 teaspoon salt

- 1/4 teaspoon ground black pepper

- 1/4 teaspoon ground nutmeg

- 1/4 teaspoon paprika

- 1/4 teaspoon dried thyme leaves

Instructions:

1. Turn on your oven and set it to 350°F (175°C) and grease a baking dish.

2. If you're using frozen corn kernels, thaw them and drain any excess liquid. If using fresh corn, cut the kernels off the cob.

3. In a large mixing bowl, beat the eggs.

4. Add the melted unsalted butter, whole milk, cornmeal, granulated sugar, salt, ground black pepper, ground nutmeg, paprika, and dried thyme leaves to the beaten eggs. Mix sufficiently until all the ingredients are thoroughly combined.

5. Stir in the fresh or thawed corn kernels, ensuring evenly distributed in the mixture.

6. Pour the corn pudding mixture into the greased baking dish.

7. Bake in the preheated oven for about 45 minutes or until the pudding is set and the top is golden brown.

8. Remove from the oven and let it cool slightly before serving.

Nutritional Information (per serving):

- Carbs: 31g

- Fats: 10g

- Fiber: 3g

- Sodium: 297mg

- Protein: 6g

Garlic Mashed Potatoes

Prep Time: 15 minutes

Cook Time: 25 minutes

Servings: 4

Ingredients:

- 4 large russet potatoes, peeled and cut into 2-inch chunks
- 4 cloves garlic, peeled
- 1/2 cup whole milk
- 3 tablespoons unsalted butter
- 1/2 teaspoon salt, or to taste
- 1/4 teaspoon ground black pepper, or to taste
- Fresh chives for garnish (optional)

Instructions:

1. Place the peeled and cut russet potatoes in a large pot. Add enough water to cover the potatoes by about an inch.

2. Add the peeled garlic cloves to the pot with the potatoes.

3. Bring the water to a boil over medium-high heat. Reduce the heat to a simmer and cook the potatoes and garlic for about 15-20 minutes, or until the potatoes are tender and easily pierced with a fork.

4. Drain the potatoes and garlic thoroughly.

5. In a small saucepan, heat the whole milk and unsalted butter over low heat until the butter is melted and the mixture is warm.

6. Using a potato masher or a fork, mash the cooked potatoes and garlic in a large mixing bowl.

7. Gradually add the warm milk and butter mixture to the mashed potatoes, mixing as you go, until you reach your desired creamy consistency.

8. Season the mashed potatoes with salt and ground black pepper, adjusting to taste.

9. Transfer the mashed potatoes to a serving dish and garnish with fresh chives, if desired.

Nutritional Information (per serving):

- Carbs: 56g

- Fats: 15g

- Fiber: 5g

- Sodium: 322mg

- Protein: 6g

Steamed Broccoli with Almonds

Prep Time: 10 minutes

Cook Time: 10 minutes

Servings: 4

Ingredients:

- 4 cups fresh broccoli florets

- 1/4 cup slivered almonds

- 2 tablespoons unsalted butter

- 1/4 teaspoon salt

- 1/8 teaspoon ground black pepper

- 1 tablespoon fresh lemon juice (optional)

Instructions:

1. Begin by preparing the fresh broccoli florets. Cut the broccoli into bite-sized pieces.

2. In a steamer basket or a microwave-safe dish, place the prepared broccoli florets.

3. Steam the broccoli until it is tender but still retains a slight crispness, about 5-7 minutes. If using a microwave, cover the dish and microwave on high for 3-4 minutes, checking for doneness.

4. While the broccoli is steaming, toast the slivered almonds in a dry skillet over medium-low heat for about 2-3 minutes, or until they become lightly golden and fragrant. Keep a close eye on them to prevent burning.

5. In a small saucepan, melt the unsalted butter over low heat.

6. Once the broccoli is steamed to your liking, remove it from the steamer or microwave and transfer it to a serving bowl.

7. Pour the melted butter over the steamed broccoli and toss to coat evenly.

8. Sprinkle the toasted slivered almonds over the broccoli and season with salt and ground black pepper.

9. If desired, drizzle fresh lemon juice over the top for added flavor.

10. Serve the Steamed Broccoli with Almonds as a delightful and gentle side dish.

Nutritional Information (per serving):

- Carbs: 7g

- Fats: 9g

- Fiber: 4g

- Sodium: 200mg

- Protein: 4g

Sautéed Spinach with Garlic

Prep Time: 5 minutes

Cook Time: 5 minutes

Servings: 4

Ingredients:

- 8 cups fresh spinach leaves, washed and stems removed

- 2 cloves garlic, minced

- 2 tablespoons olive oil

- 1/4 teaspoon salt

- 1/8 teaspoon ground black pepper

- 1/4 teaspoon red pepper flakes (optional)

Instructions:

1. Start by washing the fresh spinach leaves thoroughly and removing any tough stems.

2. In a large skillet, heat the olive oil over medium-low heat.

3. Add the minced garlic to the skillet and sauté for about 30 seconds to 1 minute, or until it becomes fragrant. Be careful not to let it brown.

4. Add the fresh spinach leaves to the skillet in batches, if necessary, as they wilt down when cooked.

5. Gently toss the spinach in the olive oil and garlic mixture. Cook for 2-3 minutes, or until the spinach is just wilted but still vibrant green.

6. Season the sautéed spinach with salt, ground black pepper, and red pepper flakes (if using). Toss to coat evenly.

7. Take out the skillet from the heat.

8. Serve the Sautéed Spinach with Garlic as a nutritious and gastroparesis-friendly side dish.

Nutritional Information (per serving):

- Carbs: 2g

- Fats: 7g

- Fiber: 2g

- Sodium: 176mg

- Protein: 2g

Roasted Carrots with Dill

Prep Time: 10 minutes

Cook Time: 25 minutes

Servings: 4

Ingredients:

- 1 pound fresh carrots, peeled and cut into sticks

- 2 tablespoons olive oil
- 1/2 teaspoon salt
- 1/4 teaspoon ground black pepper
- 1 tablespoon fresh dill, finely chopped
- 1/2 lemon, juiced

Instructions:

1. Turn on your oven and set it to 425°F (220°C).
2. Peel the fresh carrots and cut them into sticks or strips.
3. In a large mixing bowl, toss the carrot sticks with olive oil, ensuring evenly coated.
4. Season the carrots with salt and ground black pepper. Toss again to distribute the seasoning evenly.
5. Spread the seasoned carrot sticks in a single layer on a baking sheet.
6. Roast the carrots in the preheated oven for about 20-25 minutes, or until tender and slightly caramelized, stirring once halfway through the cooking time.
7. While the carrots are still hot, sprinkle the freshly chopped dill over them and drizzle with the juice of half a lemon. Toss to combine, allowing the flavors to meld.
8. Transfer the Roasted Carrots with Dill to a serving dish and garnish with additional dill, if desired.

Nutritional Information (per serving):

- Carbs: 9g
- Fats: 7g
- Fiber: 3g
- Sodium: 312mg
- Protein: 1g

Mashed Cauliflower with Chives

Prep Time: 10 minutes

Cook Time: 20 minutes

Servings: 4

Ingredients:

- 1 large head of cauliflower, chopped into florets
- 2 tablespoons unsalted butter
- 2 tablespoons fresh chives, finely chopped
- 1/4 teaspoon salt
- 1/8 teaspoon ground black pepper
- 1/4 cup whole milk

Instructions:

1. Start by chopping the large head of cauliflower into florets. Discard the tough stem.

2. Place the cauliflower florets in a large pot and add enough water to cover them.

3. Bring the water to a boil over medium-high heat, then reduce the heat to medium and let the cauliflower simmer for about 10-12 minutes, or until it is tender when pierced with a fork.

4. Drain the cooked cauliflower thoroughly.

5. In the same pot or a mixing bowl, add the drained cauliflower, unsalted butter, finely chopped chives, salt, and ground black pepper.

6. Use a potato masher or a fork to mash the cauliflower until it reaches your desired consistency. You can leave some texture or make it smooth, depending on your preference.

7. Gradually add the whole milk while continuing to mash the cauliflower. Mix sufficiently until the mashed cauliflower is creamy and well combined.

8. Taste the Mashed Cauliflower with Chives and adjust the seasoning, adding more salt or ground black pepper if needed.

9. Serve the mashed cauliflower as a delicious and gastroparesis-friendly side dish.

Nutritional Information (per serving):

- Carbs: 8g
- Fats: 4g
- Fiber: 4g
- Sodium: 179mg
- Protein: 3g

Ginger Glazed Carrots

Prep Time: 10 minutes

Cook Time: 20 minutes

Servings: 4

Ingredients:

- 1 pound fresh carrots, peeled and sliced into coins
- 2 tablespoons unsalted butter
- 2 tablespoons honey
- 1 teaspoon fresh ginger, grated
- 1/4 teaspoon salt
- 1/8 teaspoon ground black pepper
- 1/4 cup water
- Fresh parsley for garnish (optional)

Instructions:

1. Begin by peeling the fresh carrots and slicing them into coins.
2. In a large skillet or frying pan, melt the unsalted butter over medium heat.
3. Add the sliced carrots to the skillet and sauté for about 5 minutes, or until they start to become tender.

4. In a small bowl, add the honey, grated fresh ginger, salt, and ground black pepper.

5. Pour the honey and ginger mixture over the sautéed carrots and toss to coat them evenly.

6. Add the water to the skillet and stir sufficiently. This will help create a glaze for the carrots.

7. Reduce the heat to low, cover the skillet, and let the carrots simmer for about 10-15 minutes, or until tender and the glaze has thickened.

8. Stir the carrots occasionally during the simmering process to ensure evenly coated with the glaze.

9. Once the carrots are tender and the glaze has thickened, take them out from the heat.

10. Serve the Ginger Glazed Carrots as a delightful and gastroparesis-friendly side dish. Garnish with fresh parsley if desired.

Nutritional Information (per serving):

- Carbs: 24g

- Fats: 5g

- Fiber: 3g

- Sodium: 194mg

- Protein: 1g

Lemon Herb Quinoa

Prep Time: 15 minutes

Cook Time: 15 minutes

Servings: 4

Ingredients:

- 1 cup quinoa

- 2 cups water

- Zest and juice of 1 lemon
- 2 tablespoons olive oil
- 1/4 cup fresh parsley, finely chopped
- 1/4 cup fresh mint, finely chopped
- 1/4 teaspoon salt
- 1/8 teaspoon ground black pepper
- 1/4 cup cucumber, finely diced
- 1/4 cup red bell pepper, finely diced
- 1/4 cup cherry tomatoes, quartered
- 1/4 cup crumbled feta cheese (optional)

Instructions:

1. Begin by rinsing the quinoa thoroughly under cold water using a fine-mesh sieve.

2. In a medium saucepan, bring two cups of water to a boil. Add the rinsed quinoa and reduce the heat to low. Cover and simmer for about 12-15 minutes, or until the quinoa is cooked and the water is absorbed.

3. While the quinoa is cooking, prepare the dressing. In a small bowl, whisk the lemon zest, lemon juice, olive oil, finely chopped parsley, finely chopped mint, salt, and ground black pepper. Set aside.

4. Once the quinoa is cooked, fluff it with a fork and let it cool to room temperature.

5. In a large mixing bowl, add the cooked quinoa, finely diced cucumber, finely diced red bell pepper, and quartered cherry tomatoes.

6. Pour the prepared lemon herb dressing over the quinoa and vegetables. Toss well to coat all the ingredients evenly.

7. If desired, sprinkle crumbled feta cheese on top of the salad.

8. Serve the Lemon Herb Quinoa chilled or at room temperature.

Nutritional Information (per serving):

- Carbohydrates: 34g

- Fats: 9g

- Fiber: 4g

- Sodium: 191mg

- Protein: 7g

Sliced Cucumber with Yogurt Dill Sauce

Prep Time: 10 minutes

Cook Time: 0 minutes

Servings: 4

Ingredients:

- 2 large cucumbers, thinly sliced

- 1 cup plain yogurt

- 1 tablespoon fresh dill, finely chopped

- 1 clove garlic, minced

- 1/4 teaspoon salt

- 1/8 teaspoon ground black pepper

- 1 tablespoon olive oil

Instructions:

1. Begin by washing the cucumbers thoroughly and then thinly slicing them. You can leave the skin on or peel them, depending on your preference.

2. In a mixing bowl, add the plain yogurt, finely chopped fresh dill, minced garlic, salt, and ground black pepper. Mix sufficiently to create the yogurt dill sauce.

3. Place the sliced cucumbers in a serving dish.

4. Drizzle the olive oil over the sliced cucumbers.

5. Pour the prepared yogurt dill sauce over the cucumbers.

6. Gently toss the cucumber slices to coat them evenly with the yogurt dill sauce.

7. Serve the Sliced Cucumber with Yogurt Dill Sauce as a refreshing and gastroparesis-friendly side dish.

Nutritional Information (per serving):

- Carbohydrates: 9g

- Fats: 6g

- Fiber: 1g

- Sodium: 224mg

- Protein: 3g

SNACKS

Baked Cinnamon Apple Slices
Prep Time: 15 minutes
Cook Time: 25 minutes
Number of Servings: 4

Ingredients:

- 4 medium-sized apples, peeled, cored, and thinly sliced

- 2 tablespoons unsalted butter, melted

- 1/4 cup brown sugar

- 1 teaspoon ground cinnamon

- 1/4 teaspoon salt

Instructions:

1. Turn on your oven and set it to 350°F (175°C).

2. In a medium-sized bowl, add the thinly sliced apples, melted unsalted butter, brown sugar, ground cinnamon, and salt. Toss the ingredients together until the apple slices are evenly coated.

3. Place the coated apple slices in a single layer in a baking dish.

4. Bake in the preheated oven for approximately 25 minutes, or until the apple slices are tender and have a slight caramelized appearance.

5. Take out the baked cinnamon apple slices from the oven and let them cool for a few minutes before serving.

Nutritional Information (per serving):

- Carbs: 34 grams

- Fats: 6 grams

- Fiber: 5 grams

- Sodium: 75 milligrams

- Protein: 0 grams

Rice Cakes with Cottage Cheese and Berries

Prep Time: 10 minutes
Cook Time: None
Number of Servings: 2

Ingredients:

- 4 rice cakes

- 1 cup low-fat cottage cheese

- 1/2 cup fresh berries (e.g., strawberries, blueberries, or raspberries)

- 1 tablespoon honey

- 1/4 teaspoon ground cinnamon

Instructions:

1. Take the 4 rice cakes and place them on a clean surface or plate.

2. Spread an equal amount of low-fat cottage cheese (1/2 cup each) evenly over each rice cake.

3. Wash and prepare the fresh berries of your choice (e.g., strawberries, blueberries, or raspberries). If using strawberries, take out the stems and slice them.

4. Top each cottage cheese-covered rice cake with your prepared berries. Distribute them evenly.

5. Drizzle 1/2 tablespoon of honey over each rice cake with berries.

6. Finish by sprinkling a pinch (about 1/8 teaspoon) of ground cinnamon over each rice cake.

7. Your Rice Cakes with Cottage Cheese and Berries are ready to be enjoyed!

Nutritional Information (per serving):

- Carbs: 26 grams

- Fats: 2 grams

- Fiber: 3 grams

- Sodium: 280 milligrams

- Protein: 13 grams

Roasted Pumpkin Seeds with Sea Salt

Prep Time: 10 minutes
Cook Time: 30 minutes
Number of Servings: 4

Ingredients:

- 2 cups pumpkin seeds, cleaned and dried

- 2 teaspoons olive oil

- 1/2 teaspoon sea salt

Instructions:

1. Turn on your oven and set it to 300°F (150°C).

2. In a mixing bowl, add the cleaned and dried pumpkin seeds with two teaspoons of olive oil. Toss the seeds until evenly coated.

3. Spread the coated pumpkin seeds in a single layer on a baking sheet.

4. Sprinkle 1/2 teaspoon of sea salt evenly over the pumpkin seeds.

5. Place the baking sheet in the preheated oven and roast the seeds for approximately 30 minutes, or until golden brown and crispy. Be sure to stir the seeds every 10 minutes to ensure even roasting.

6. Once roasted to your desired level of crispiness, take out the pumpkin seeds from the oven and let them cool on the baking sheet.

7. Once cooled, transfer the Roasted Pumpkin Seeds with Sea Salt to an airtight container for storage or enjoy them as a snack.

Nutritional Information (per serving):

- Carbs: 4 grams

- Fats: 13 grams

- Fiber: 2 grams

- Sodium: 292 milligrams

- Protein: 7 grams

Peach and Banana Smoothie

Prep Time: 10 minutes
Cook Time: None
Number of Servings: 2

Ingredients:

- 2 ripe peaches, pitted and sliced

- 2 ripe bananas, peeled and sliced

- 1 cup lactose-free yogurt

- 1/2 cup unsweetened almond milk

- 1 tablespoon honey (optional)

- Ice cubes (optional)

Instructions:

1. Prepare the peaches by washing, pitting, and slicing them.

2. Peel the ripe bananas and slice them.

3. In a blender, add the sliced peaches, sliced bananas, lactose-free yogurt, unsweetened almond milk, and optional honey.

4. Blend the ingredients on high speed until smooth and creamy. If a thicker consistency is desired, add a few ice cubes and blend again.

5. Pour the Peach and Banana Smoothie into glasses for serving.

6. Garnish with additional slices of peach or banana if desired.

7. Serve immediately and enjoy this refreshing smoothie!

Nutritional Information (per serving):

- Carbs: 48 grams

- Fats: 4 grams

- Fiber: 6 grams

- Sodium: 62 milligrams

- Protein: 5 grams

Greek Yogurt Parfait with Kiwi
Prep Time: 10 minutes
Cook Time: None
Number of Servings: 2

Ingredients:

- 1 cup low-fat Greek yogurt

- 2 ripe kiwis, peeled and diced

- 1/4 cup gluten-free granola

- 1 tablespoon honey (optional)

Instructions:

1. In a bowl, scoop out one cup of low-fat Greek yogurt.

2. Peel the ripe kiwis and dice them into small pieces.

3. In serving glasses or bowls, start by layering the Greek yogurt. Divide it equally between the two servings.

4. Add the diced kiwi on top of the Greek yogurt in each glass.

5. Sprinkle two tablespoons of gluten-free granola over the kiwi layer in each serving.

6. If desired, drizzle 1/2 tablespoon of honey over each parfait for added sweetness.

7. Your Greek Yogurt Parfait with Kiwi is ready to be enjoyed!

Nutritional Information (per serving):

- Carbs: 35 grams

- Fats: 2 grams

- Fiber: 4 grams

- Sodium: 65 milligrams

- Protein: 10 grams

Almond Flour Banana Muffins

Prep Time: 15 minutes
Cook Time: 25 minutes
Number of Servings: 12 muffins

Ingredients:

- 2 cups almond flour

- 1/4 cup coconut flour

- 1 teaspoon baking soda

- 1/4 teaspoon salt

- 3 ripe bananas, mashed

- 3 large eggs

- 1/4 cup coconut oil, melted

- 1/4 cup pure maple syrup

- 1 teaspoon pure vanilla extract

- 1/2 cup chopped walnuts (optional)

Instructions:

1. Turn on your oven and set it to 350°F (175°C). Grease or line a muffin tin with paper liners.

2. In a mixing bowl, add two cups of almond flour, 1/4 cup of coconut flour, one teaspoon of baking soda, and 1/4 teaspoon of salt.

3. In another bowl, mash the 3 ripe bananas until smooth.

4. Add 3 large eggs, 1/4 cup of melted coconut oil, 1/4 cup of pure maple syrup, and one teaspoon of pure vanilla extract to the

mashed bananas. Mix sufficiently until all the wet ingredients are fully combined.

5. Pour the wet ingredients into the dry ingredients and stir until a uniform batter forms.

6. If using, fold in 1/2 cup of chopped walnuts.

7. Spoon the batter evenly into the prepared muffin tin, filling each cup about 2/3 full.

8. Bake in the preheated oven for approximately 25 minutes, or until the muffins are golden brown and a toothpick inserted into the center comes out clean.

9. Take out the muffins from the oven and let them cool in the muffin tin for a few minutes before transferring them to a wire rack to cool completely.

10. Once cooled, your Almond Flour Banana Muffins are ready to be enjoyed!

Nutritional Information (per muffin):

- Carbs: 14 grams

- Fats: 13 grams

- Fiber: 3 grams

- Sodium: 171 milligrams

- Protein: 5 grams

Cucumber and Bell Pepper Sticks with Hummus

Prep Time: 10 minutes
Cook Time: None
Number of Servings: 4

Ingredients:

- 2 large cucumbers, peeled and cut into sticks

- 2 large bell peppers (red, yellow, or green), cut into sticks

- 1 cup hummus

- Fresh parsley leaves for garnish (optional)

Instructions:

1. Start by preparing the cucumbers. Peel them and then cut them into sticks.

2. Prepare the bell peppers by cutting them into sticks as well.

3. Arrange the cucumber and bell pepper sticks on a serving platter.

4. In a separate bowl, place one cup of hummus for dipping.

5. If desired, garnish the platter with fresh parsley leaves for a touch of color.

6. Serve the Cucumber and Bell Pepper Sticks with Hummus as a healthy and refreshing snack.

Nutritional Information (per serving):

- Carbs: 20 grams

- Fats: 6 grams

- Fiber: 6 grams

- Sodium: 190 milligrams

- Protein: 5 grams

Baked Sweet Potato Fries

Prep Time: 15 minutes
Cook Time: 25 minutes
Number of Servings: 4

Ingredients:

- 4 medium-sized sweet potatoes, peeled and cut into fries

- 2 tablespoons olive oil

- 1/2 teaspoon salt

- 1/4 teaspoon black pepper

- 1/4 teaspoon paprika (optional)

- 1/4 teaspoon garlic powder (optional)

Instructions:

1. Turn on your oven and set it to 425°F (220°C).

2. Peel the 4 medium-sized sweet potatoes and cut them into fries.

3. In a large mixing bowl, add the sweet potato fries with two tablespoons of olive oil. Toss to coat the fries evenly with the oil.

4. Season the fries with 1/2 teaspoon of salt, 1/4 teaspoon of black pepper, and optionally, 1/4 teaspoon of paprika and 1/4 teaspoon of garlic powder for added flavor.

5. Spread the seasoned sweet potato fries in a single layer on a baking sheet.

6. Bake in the preheated oven for approximately 25 minutes, or until the fries are golden brown and crispy, turning them over halfway through the cooking time for even browning.

7. Once done, take out the Baked Sweet Potato Fries from the oven and serve immediately.

Nutritional Information (per serving):

- Carbs: 30 grams

- Fats: 5 grams

- Fiber: 4 grams

- Sodium: 340 milligrams

- Protein: 2 grams

Cheddar Cheese Slices with Sliced Pear

Prep Time: 10 minutes
Cook Time: None
Number of Servings: 2

Ingredients:

- 4 slices of cheddar cheese

- 1 ripe pear, thinly sliced

- Fresh lemon juice (from 1/2 lemon)
- Freshly ground black pepper, to taste

Instructions:

1. Begin by slicing 1 ripe pear into thin slices.
2. Squeeze the juice from 1/2 lemon over the pear slices to prevent browning and add a refreshing touch.
3. Arrange 4 slices of cheddar cheese on a serving platter.
4. Place the thinly sliced pear on top of the cheddar cheese slices.
5. Finish by adding freshly ground black pepper to taste for a hint of spice.
6. Serve the Cheddar Cheese Slices with Sliced Pear as a light and delicious snack or appetizer.

Nutritional Information (per serving):

- Carbs: 15 grams
- Fats: 16 grams
- Fiber: 3 grams
- Sodium: 400 milligrams
- Protein: 11 grams

Watermelon and Mint Skewers

Prep Time: 15 minutes
Cook Time: None
Number of Servings: 4

Ingredients:

- 2 cups watermelon, diced into 1-inch cubes
- 16 fresh mint leaves
- 4 wooden skewers

Instructions:

1. Begin by preparing the watermelon. Cut it into 1-inch cubes, resulting in approximately two cups of diced watermelon.

2. Wash and pat dry 16 fresh mint leaves.

3. Take 4 wooden skewers and assemble the Watermelon and Mint Skewers by threading diced watermelon and mint leaves alternately onto each skewer.

4. Continue this pattern until each skewer has a colorful and refreshing arrangement of watermelon and mint.

5. Serve the Watermelon and Mint Skewers immediately as a delightful and hydrating snack.

Nutritional Information (per serving):

- Carbs: 9 grams

- Fats: 0 grams

- Fiber: 1 gram

- Sodium: 2 milligrams

- Protein: 0 grams

Rice Cakes with Almond Butter

Prep Time: 5 minutes
Cook Time: None
Number of Servings: 2

Ingredients:

- 4 rice cakes

- 4 tablespoons almond butter

- 2 teaspoons honey (optional)

Instructions:

1. Take 4 rice cakes and place them on a clean surface or plate.

2. Spread two tablespoons of almond butter evenly over each rice cake.

3. If desired, drizzle one teaspoon of honey over each almond butter-covered rice cake for added sweetness.

4. Your Rice Cakes with Almond Butter are ready to be enjoyed!

Nutritional Information (per serving):

- Carbs: 26 grams

- Fats: 14 grams

- Fiber: 2 grams

- Sodium: 115 milligrams

- Protein: 7 grams

Banana and Peanut Butter Smoothie

Prep Time: 5 minutes
Cook Time: None
Number of Servings: 2

Ingredients:

- 2 ripe bananas

- 4 tablespoons natural peanut butter

- 1 cup lactose-free yogurt

- 1/2 cup unsweetened almond milk

- 1 teaspoon honey (optional)

- Ice cubes (optional)

Instructions:

1. Peel and slice 2 ripe bananas.

2. In a blender, add the sliced bananas, 4 tablespoons of natural peanut butter, one cup of lactose-free yogurt, and 1/2 cup of unsweetened almond milk.

3. If you desire added sweetness, add one teaspoon of honey to the blender.

4. For a colder and thicker smoothie, consider adding a few ice cubes to the blender.

5. Blend all the ingredients together on high speed until you achieve a smooth and creamy consistency.

6. Once blended to your satisfaction, pour the Banana and Peanut Butter Smoothie into glasses for serving.

7. Serve immediately and enjoy this delicious and nourishing smoothie!

Nutritional Information (per serving):

- Carbs: 30 grams

- Fats: 17 grams

- Fiber: 4 grams

- Sodium: 200 milligrams

- Protein: 11 grams

Roasted Chickpeas with Paprika

Prep Time: 10 minutes
Cook Time: 30 minutes
Number of Servings: 4

Ingredients:

- 2 cans (15 ounces each) of canned chickpeas, drained and rinsed

- 2 tablespoons olive oil

- 1 teaspoon paprika

- 1/2 teaspoon salt

- 1/4 teaspoon black pepper

- 1/4 teaspoon garlic powder (optional)

Instructions:

1. Turn on your oven and set it to 400°F (200°C).

2. Drain and rinse 2 cans of chickpeas. Pat them dry with a clean kitchen towel or paper towels to remove excess moisture.

3. In a bowl, add the dried chickpeas with two tablespoons of olive oil. Toss them until evenly coated with the oil.

4. Season the chickpeas with one teaspoon of paprika, 1/2 teaspoon of salt, 1/4 teaspoon of black pepper, and optionally, 1/4 teaspoon of garlic powder for added flavor.

5. Spread the seasoned chickpeas in a single layer on a baking sheet.

6. Roast the chickpeas in the preheated oven for approximately 30 minutes, or until crispy and golden brown. Stir them or shake the pan every 10 minutes for even roasting.

7. Once done, take out the Roasted Chickpeas with Paprika from the oven and let them cool slightly before serving.

8. Enjoy these crunchy and flavorful chickpeas as a delicious and gastroparesis-friendly snack!

Nutritional Information (per serving):

- Carbs: 21 grams

- Fats: 7 grams

- Fiber: 6 grams

- Sodium: 385 milligrams

- Protein: 7 grams

Cottage Cheese with Pineapple

Prep Time: 5 minutes
Cook Time: None
Number of Servings: 2

Ingredients:

- 1 cup low-fat cottage cheese

- 1 cup fresh pineapple chunks

- 1 tablespoon honey (optional)

Instructions:

1. Start by preparing one cup of low-fat cottage cheese.

2. Cut one cup of fresh pineapple into small chunks.

3. In serving bowls, place 1/2 cup of the prepared low-fat cottage cheese in each bowl.

4. Add 1/2 cup of the fresh pineapple chunks on top of the cottage cheese in each bowl.

5. If desired, drizzle 1/2 tablespoon of honey over each serving for added sweetness.

6. Your Cottage Cheese with Pineapple is ready to be enjoyed as a light and refreshing snack or breakfast option.

Nutritional Information (per serving):

- Carbs: 24 grams

- Fats: 2 grams

- Fiber: 2 grams

- Sodium: 440 milligrams

- Protein: 15 grams

Greek Yogurt with Honey and Berries

Prep Time: 5 minutes
Cook Time: None
Number of Servings: 2

Ingredients:

- 2 cups lactose-free Greek yogurt

- 1/2 cup fresh mixed berries (e.g., strawberries, blueberries, raspberries)

- 2 tablespoons honey (optional)

Instructions:

1. Begin by scooping out two cups of lactose-free Greek yogurt.

2. Wash and prepare 1/2 cup of fresh mixed berries, such as strawberries, blueberries, and raspberries.

3. In serving bowls, place one cup of the lactose-free Greek yogurt in each bowl.

4. Top the Greek yogurt in each bowl with 1/4 cup of the prepared mixed berries.

5. If desired, drizzle one tablespoon of honey over each serving for added sweetness.

6. Your Greek Yogurt with Honey and Berries is ready to be enjoyed as a delicious and gastroparesis-friendly snack or breakfast.

Nutritional Information (per serving):

- Carbs: 34 grams

- Fats: 1 gram

- Fiber: 2 grams

- Sodium: 110 milligrams

- Protein: 17 grams

Baked Apple Chips

Prep Time: 15 minutes
Cook Time: 2-3 hours
Number of Servings: 4

Ingredients:

- 4 medium-sized apples

- 1 teaspoon ground cinnamon

- 1/2 teaspoon granulated sugar (optional)

Instructions:

1. Turn on your oven and set it to 225°F (110°C). Line two baking sheets with parchment paper or silicone baking mats.

2. Wash and core 4 medium-sized apples. Leave the skin on for added fiber.

3. Using a sharp knife or a mandoline slicer, slice the apples into very thin, even rounds. Aim for slices that are about 1/8 inch thick.

4. In a large bowl, add the apple slices with one teaspoon of ground cinnamon. If you prefer a slightly sweeter flavor, you can add 1/2 teaspoon of granulated sugar, but this is optional.

5. Arrange the cinnamon-coated apple slices in a single layer on the prepared baking sheets. Make sure not overlapping to ensure even baking.

6. Place the baking sheets in the preheated oven and bake the apple slices for 2-3 hours. Check them occasionally and flip the slices over to ensure they dry out evenly.

7. Take out the Baked Apple Chips from the oven when crisp and have a golden-brown color. The exact time may vary depending on your oven and the thickness of the slices.

8. Allow the apple chips to cool completely on the baking sheets. They will continue to crisp up as they cool.

9. Once cooled, transfer the Baked Apple Chips to an airtight container for storage.

10. Enjoy these gastroparesis-friendly Baked Apple Chips as a healthy and satisfying snack!

Nutritional Information (per serving):

- Carbs: 24 grams

- Fats: 0 grams

- Fiber: 5 grams

- Sodium: 1 milligram

- Protein: 0 grams

Carrot and Celery Sticks with Hummus

Prep Time: 10 minutes
Cook Time: None
Number of Servings: 4

Ingredients:

- 4 large carrots, peeled and cut into sticks

- 4 celery stalks, cut into sticks

- 1 cup hummus

- Fresh parsley leaves for garnish (optional)

Instructions:

1. Begin by preparing the carrots. Peel them and then cut them into sticks.

2. Cut 4 celery stalks into sticks as well.

3. Arrange the carrot and celery sticks on a serving platter.

4. In a separate bowl, place one cup of hummus for dipping.

5. If desired, garnish the platter with fresh parsley leaves for a touch of color.

6. Serve the Carrot and Celery Sticks with Hummus as a healthy and refreshing snack or appetizer.

Nutritional Information (per serving):

- Carbs: 21 grams

- Fats: 5 grams

- Fiber: 6 grams

- Sodium: 395 milligrams

- Protein: 7 grams

Boiled Edamame with Sea Salt

Prep Time: 5 minutes
Cook Time: 5 minutes
Number of Servings: 4

Ingredients:

- 2 cups frozen edamame in pods

- 1 tablespoon sea salt

Instructions:

1. Start by bringing a pot of water to a boil. You'll need enough water to submerge two cups of frozen edamame.

2. While the water is heating, prepare the edamame. If using frozen edamame, there's no need to thaw them; you can cook them directly from frozen.

3. Once the water is boiling, add one tablespoon of sea salt to the boiling water.

4. Carefully add the frozen edamame pods to the boiling water.

5. Allow the edamame to boil for about 5 minutes. Keep an eye on them, as they can overcook quickly.

6. After 5 minutes, use a slotted spoon to scoop the boiled edamame out of the water and into a serving bowl.

7. Sprinkle a bit more sea salt over the boiled edamame if desired, for extra flavor.

8. Serve the Boiled Edamame with Sea Salt as a simple and gastroparesis-friendly snack or appetizer.

Nutritional Information (per serving):

- Carbs: 9 grams

- Fats: 2 grams

- Fiber: 5 grams

- Sodium: 880 milligrams

- Protein: 8 grams

155

DESSERTS

Almond Flour Chocolate Chip Cookies
Prep Time: 15 minutes
Cook Time: 12 minutes
Number of Servings: 12 cookies

Ingredients:

- 2 cups almond flour
- 1/2 cup coconut oil (melted)
- 1/4 cup honey
- 1/4 cup dark chocolate chips
- 1/4 cup unsweetened shredded coconut
- 1/4 teaspoon baking soda
- 1/4 teaspoon salt
- 1 teaspoon vanilla extract

Instructions:

1. Turn on your oven and set it to 350°F (180°C) and line a baking sheet with parchment paper.

2. In a mixing bowl, add two cups of almond flour, 1/4 teaspoon of baking soda, and 1/4 teaspoon of salt.

3. In a separate microwave-safe bowl, melt 1/2 cup of coconut oil. This usually takes about 30 seconds in the microwave.

4. Add 1/4 cup of honey and one teaspoon of vanilla extract to the melted coconut oil. Stir sufficiently to combine.

5. Pour the wet mixture into the dry ingredients and mix until you have a uniform cookie dough.

6. Gently fold in 1/4 cup of dark chocolate chips and 1/4 cup of unsweetened shredded coconut into the dough.

7. Using a cookie scoop or spoon, drop spoonfuls of cookie dough onto the prepared baking sheet, spacing them about 2 inches apart.

8. Flatten each cookie slightly with the back of a spoon or your fingers.

9. Bake in the preheated oven for 10-12 minutes or until the cookies turn golden brown around the edges.

10. Take out the cookies from the oven and allow them to cool on the baking sheet for a few minutes before transferring them to a wire rack to cool completely.

Nutritional Information (Per Serving):

- Carbohydrates: 12g

- Fats: 18g

- Fiber: 2g

- Sodium: 75mg

- Protein: 3g

Chia Seed and Coconut Pudding

Prep Time: 5 minutes
Cook Time: 0 minutes
Number of Servings: 4 servings

Ingredients:

- 1/2 cup chia seeds

- 2 cups unsweetened coconut milk

- 2 tablespoons honey

- 1/4 cup shredded coconut (unsweetened)

- 1/4 teaspoon vanilla extract

- Fresh berries for garnish (optional)

Instructions:

1. In a mixing bowl, add 1/2 cup of chia seeds, two cups of unsweetened coconut milk, two tablespoons of honey, 1/4 cup of shredded coconut, and 1/4 teaspoon of vanilla extract.

2. Stir the mixture well until all ingredients are fully combined. Make sure the chia seeds are evenly distributed.

3. Cover the bowl and refrigerate the mixture for at least 2 hours or overnight. This will allow the chia seeds to absorb the liquid and thicken the pudding.

4. Before serving, give the pudding a good stir to redistribute the chia seeds evenly.

5. Divide the chia seed and coconut pudding into 4 serving cups or bowls.

6. If desired, garnish with fresh berries.

7. Serve chilled and enjoy!

Nutritional Information (Per Serving):

- Carbohydrates: 17g

- Fats: 14g

- Fiber: 9g

- Sodium: 15mg

- Protein: 4g

Baked Cinnamon Pears

Prep Time: 10 minutes
Cook Time: 30 minutes
Number of Servings: 4 servings

Ingredients:

- 4 ripe pears

- 2 tablespoons honey

- 1 teaspoon ground cinnamon

- 1/4 cup chopped walnuts (optional)

- 1/4 cup rolled oats (gluten-free if needed)

- 1 tablespoon unsalted butter (or dairy-free alternative)

- Pinch of salt

Instructions:

1. Turn on your oven and set it to 375°F (190°C).

2. Wash and peel the 4 ripe pears. Cut them in half lengthwise and take out the cores. Place the pear halves in a baking dish, cut side up.

3. In a small bowl, add two tablespoons of honey and one teaspoon of ground cinnamon. Mix sufficiently to create a cinnamon-honey glaze.

4. Drizzle the cinnamon-honey glaze over the pear halves, ensuring each one is coated evenly.

5. In a separate bowl, add 1/4 cup of chopped walnuts (if using), 1/4 cup of rolled oats, one tablespoon of unsalted butter (or dairy-free alternative), and a pinch of salt. Mix until the ingredients are well combined.

6. Spoon the walnut and oat mixture evenly onto each pear half.

7. Cover the baking dish with aluminum foil and bake in the preheated oven for 20 minutes.

8. After 20 minutes, take out the foil and bake for an extra 10 minutes or until the pears are tender and the topping is golden brown.

9. Remove from the oven and let cool slightly before serving.

10. Serve the baked cinnamon pears warm, optionally with a dollop of yogurt or a scoop of vanilla ice cream for added richness.

Nutritional Information (Per Serving):

- Carbohydrates: 34g

- Fats: 9g

- Fiber: 6g

- Sodium: 27mg

- Protein: 2g

Chocolate Avocado Brownies (Gluten-Free)

Prep Time: 15 minutes
Cook Time: 25 minutes
Number of Servings: 12 brownies

Ingredients:

- 2 ripe avocados, mashed

- 1/2 cup unsweetened cocoa powder

- 1/2 cup honey

- 2 large eggs

- 1 teaspoon vanilla extract

- 1/2 cup almond flour

- 1/4 cup unsweetened almond butter

- 1/4 teaspoon baking soda

- Pinch of salt

- 1/2 cup dark chocolate chips

Instructions:

1. Turn on your oven and set it to 350°F (180°C). Grease an 8x8-inch (20x20 cm) baking pan and line it with parchment paper for easy removal.

2. In a bowl, mash 2 ripe avocados until smooth.

3. Add 1/2 cup of unsweetened cocoa powder to the mashed avocados. Mix until well combined.

4. Stir in 1/2 cup of honey, 2 large eggs, and one teaspoon of vanilla extract, mixing until the batter is smooth and glossy.

5. In a separate bowl, add 1/2 cup of almond flour, 1/4 cup of unsweetened almond butter, 1/4 teaspoon of baking soda, and a pinch of salt. Mix until it forms a crumbly texture.

6. Gradually add the dry mixture to the avocado mixture and stir until fully incorporated.

7. Fold in 1/2 cup of dark chocolate chips.

8. Pour the brownie batter into the prepared baking pan and spread it evenly.

9. Bake in the preheated oven for approximately 25 minutes, or until a toothpick inserted into the center comes out with a few moist crumbs.

10. Take out the brownies from the oven and let them cool in the pan for about 10 minutes.

11. Use the parchment paper overhang to lift the brownies out of the pan and onto a wire rack to cool completely.

12. Once cooled, slice into 12 squares and enjoy!

Nutritional Information (Per Serving):

- Carbohydrates: 20g

- Fats: 13g

- Fiber: 4g

- Sodium: 49mg

- Protein: 3g

Coconut Rice Pudding with Mango

Prep Time: 10 minutes
Cook Time: 30 minutes
Number of Servings: 4 servings

Ingredients:

- 1 cup Arborio rice

- 2 cups unsweetened coconut milk

- 1/4 cup honey

- 1/2 teaspoon ground cinnamon

- 1/4 teaspoon salt

- 1 teaspoon vanilla extract

- 1 ripe mango, diced

- Toasted coconut flakes for garnish (optional)

Instructions:

1. In a medium-sized saucepan, add one cup of Arborio rice, two cups of unsweetened coconut milk, 1/4 cup of honey, 1/2 teaspoon of ground cinnamon, and 1/4 teaspoon of salt.

2. Place the saucepan over medium heat and bring the mixture to a gentle simmer, stirring frequently.

3. Once it starts simmering, reduce the heat to low, cover, and let the rice cook for approximately 20-25 minutes, or until the rice is tender and the mixture has thickened, stirring occasionally.

4. Take out the saucepan from the heat and stir in one teaspoon of vanilla extract.

5. Allow the coconut rice pudding to cool slightly.

6. While the pudding is cooling, dice 1 ripe mango into small pieces.

7. To serve, spoon the coconut rice pudding into individual serving bowls and top with the diced mango.

8. If desired, garnish with toasted coconut flakes for added texture and flavor.

9. Serve the Coconut Rice Pudding with Mango warm or chilled, according to your preference.

Nutritional Information (Per Serving):

- Carbohydrates: 53g

- Fats: 12g

- Fiber: 2g

- Sodium: 160mg

- Protein: 3g

Lemon Sorbet

Prep Time: 10 minutes
Cook Time: 0 minutes
Number of Servings: 4 servings

Ingredients:

- 1 cup freshly squeezed lemon juice (from about 4-6 lemons)
- 1 cup water
- 1/2 cup honey
- Zest of 1 lemon
- Pinch of salt
- Lemon slices and fresh mint leaves for garnish (optional)

Instructions:

1. In a mixing bowl, add one cup of freshly squeezed lemon juice (about 4-6 lemons), one cup of water, 1/2 cup of honey, the zest of 1 lemon, and a pinch of salt. Mix until the honey is completely dissolved.

2. Pour the lemon mixture into an ice cream maker.

3. Churn the mixture according to the manufacturer's instructions for your ice cream maker. This usually takes about 20-25 minutes.

4. Once the sorbet reaches a soft-serve consistency, transfer it to an airtight container and freeze for at least 2 hours to firm up.

5. Prior to serving, allow the sorbet to sit at room temperature for a few minutes to soften slightly for easier scooping.

6. Scoop the lemon sorbet into bowls or serving dishes.

7. Garnish with lemon slices and fresh mint leaves if desired.

8. Serve the refreshing Lemon Sorbet immediately.

Nutritional Information (Per Serving):

- Carbohydrates: 35g

- Fats: 0g

- Fiber: 0g

- Sodium: 26mg

- Protein: 0g

Vanilla Almond Milkshake

Prep Time: 5 minutes
Cook Time: 0 minutes
Number of Servings: 2 servings

Ingredients:

- 2 cups unsweetened almond milk

- 1 ripe banana, peeled and sliced

- 2 tablespoons honey

- 1 teaspoon vanilla extract

- 1/2 cup ice cubes

- Ground cinnamon for garnish (optional)

Instructions:

1. In a blender, add two cups of unsweetened almond milk, 1 ripe banana (peeled and sliced), two tablespoons of honey, and one teaspoon of vanilla extract.

2. Add 1/2 cup of ice cubes to the blender to make the milkshake cold and refreshing.

3. Blend all the ingredients on high until the mixture is smooth and creamy.

4. Taste the milkshake and adjust the sweetness if necessary by adding more honey, blending again to incorporate.

5. Once the milkshake reaches your desired level of sweetness and creaminess, stop blending.

6. Pour the vanilla almond milkshake into two glasses.

7. If desired, garnish with a sprinkle of ground cinnamon for extra flavor.

8. Serve the Vanilla Almond Milkshake immediately, using a straw or spoon to enjoy.

Nutritional Information (Per Serving):

- Carbohydrates: 27g

- Fats: 2g

- Fiber: 3g

- Sodium: 166mg

- Protein: 1g

Raspberry and Dark Chocolate Yogurt Cups

Prep Time: 15 minutes
Cook Time: 0 minutes
Number of Servings: 4 yogurt cups

Ingredients:

- 2 cups plain Greek yogurt

- 1 cup fresh raspberries

- 1/4 cup dark chocolate chips

- 2 tablespoons honey

- 1/4 teaspoon vanilla extract

- Fresh mint leaves for garnish (optional)

Instructions:

1. In a mixing bowl, add two cups of plain Greek yogurt, two tablespoons of honey, and 1/4 teaspoon of vanilla extract. Mix sufficiently until the honey and vanilla are evenly incorporated into the yogurt.

2. Wash and dry one cup of fresh raspberries.

3. In four individual serving cups or bowls, layer the yogurt mixture and raspberries. Start with a layer of yogurt, then add a few raspberries, followed by another layer of yogurt, and continue until you've used up all the ingredients. Make sure to finish with a layer of yogurt on top.

4. Place 1/4 cup of dark chocolate chips in a microwave-safe bowl. Microwave in 20-second intervals, stirring between each interval, until the chocolate chips are completely melted and smooth.

5. Drizzle the melted dark chocolate over the top of each yogurt cup.

6. If desired, garnish the Raspberry and Dark Chocolate Yogurt Cups with fresh mint leaves for a burst of color and flavor.

7. Serve the yogurt cups immediately, or refrigerate until ready to enjoy.

Nutritional Information (Per Serving):

- Carbohydrates: 29g

- Fats: 10g

- Fiber: 4g

- Sodium: 51mg

- Protein: 16g

Blueberry Crumble (Gluten-Free)

Prep Time: 15 minutes
Cook Time: 30 minutes
Number of Servings: 6 servings

Ingredients:

For the Filling:

- 4 cups fresh or frozen blueberries

- 2 tablespoons honey

- 1 tablespoon cornstarch

- 1 tablespoon lemon juice
- 1/2 teaspoon vanilla extract

For the Crumble Topping:

- 1 cup gluten-free rolled oats
- 1/2 cup almond flour
- 1/4 cup chopped nuts (e.g., almonds or walnuts)
- 1/4 cup honey
- 1/4 cup melted coconut oil (or dairy-free alternative)
- 1/2 teaspoon ground cinnamon
- Pinch of salt

Instructions:

1. Turn on your oven and set it to 350°F (180°C). Grease an 8x8-inch (20x20 cm) baking dish.

2. In a large mixing bowl, add 4 cups of fresh or frozen blueberries, two tablespoons of honey, one tablespoon of cornstarch, one tablespoon of lemon juice, and 1/2 teaspoon of vanilla extract. Toss the blueberries until well coated with the mixture.

3. In a separate bowl, prepare the crumble topping. Add one cup of gluten-free rolled oats, 1/2 cup of almond flour, 1/4 cup of chopped nuts, 1/4 cup of honey, 1/4 cup of melted coconut oil (or dairy-free alternative), 1/2 teaspoon of ground cinnamon, and a pinch of salt. Mix until the ingredients are well combined and the mixture is crumbly.

4. Pour the blueberry filling into the greased baking dish, spreading it out evenly.

5. Sprinkle the crumble topping over the blueberry filling, covering it completely.

6. Bake in the preheated oven for about 30 minutes, or until the topping is golden brown and the blueberry filling is bubbly.

7. Remove from the oven and allow the Blueberry Crumble to cool slightly before serving.

8. Serve warm as is or with a scoop of vanilla ice cream for added indulgence.

Nutritional Information (Per Serving):

- Carbohydrates: 45g

- Fats: 14g

- Fiber: 6g

- Sodium: 58mg

- Protein: 5g

Banana and Coconut Ice Cream

Prep Time: 10 minutes
Cook Time: 0 minutes
Number of Servings: 4 servings

Ingredients:

- 4 ripe bananas, peeled and sliced

- 1/2 cup unsweetened coconut milk

- 2 tablespoons honey

- 1/2 teaspoon vanilla extract

- Unsweetened shredded coconut for garnish (optional)

Instructions:

1. Slice 4 ripe bananas and place them on a baking sheet lined with parchment paper. Make sure the banana slices are not touching each other. Freeze the banana slices for at least 2 hours or until completely frozen.

2. Once the banana slices are frozen, take them out from the freezer and let them sit at room temperature for a few minutes to slightly soften, making them easier to blend.

3. In a blender, add the frozen banana slices, 1/2 cup of unsweetened coconut milk, two tablespoons of honey, and 1/2 teaspoon of vanilla extract.

4. Blend the mixture until it becomes smooth and creamy. You may need to stop and scrape down the sides of the blender a few times to ensure even blending.

5. Once the mixture is creamy and resembles ice cream, stop blending.

6. Scoop the Banana and Coconut Ice Cream into bowls or serving dishes.

7. If desired, garnish with unsweetened shredded coconut for added texture and flavor.

8. Serve the ice cream immediately. It has a soft-serve consistency right after blending.

Nutritional Information (Per Serving):

- Carbohydrates: 42g

- Fats: 4g

- Fiber: 4g

- Sodium: 4mg

- Protein: 1g

Rice Pudding with Cinnamon

Prep Time: 10 minutes
Cook Time: 30 minutes
Number of Servings: 4 servings

Ingredients:

- 1/2 cup Arborio rice

- 2 cups whole milk

- 1/4 cup honey

- 1/2 teaspoon ground cinnamon

- 1/4 teaspoon vanilla extract

- Pinch of salt

- Ground cinnamon for garnish (optional)

Instructions:

1. In a medium-sized saucepan, add 1/2 cup of Arborio rice, two cups of whole milk, 1/4 cup of honey, 1/2 teaspoon of ground cinnamon, 1/4 teaspoon of vanilla extract, and a pinch of salt.

2. Place the saucepan over medium heat and bring the mixture to a gentle simmer, stirring frequently.

3. Once it starts simmering, reduce the heat to low and let the rice pudding simmer for approximately 25-30 minutes, or until the rice is tender and the mixture has thickened, stirring occasionally.

4. Take out the saucepan from the heat and let the rice pudding cool slightly.

5. To serve, divide the Rice Pudding with Cinnamon into four individual serving bowls.

6. If desired, garnish each bowl with a sprinkle of ground cinnamon for added flavor and presentation.

7. Serve the rice pudding warm or chilled, according to your preference.

Nutritional Information (Per Serving):

- Carbohydrates: 45g

- Fats: 6g

- Fiber: 0g

- Sodium: 58mg

- Protein: 6g

Banana Ice Cream

Prep Time: 5 minutes
Cook Time: 0 minutes
Number of Servings: 2 servings

Ingredients:

- 2 ripe bananas, peeled, sliced, and frozen

- 1/4 cup unsweetened almond milk

- 1 tablespoon honey (optional)

- 1/2 teaspoon vanilla extract (optional)

- Sliced almonds for garnish (optional)

Instructions:

1. Start by slicing 2 ripe bananas and placing the banana slices in an airtight container. Freeze the banana slices for at least 2 hours or until completely frozen.

2. Once the banana slices are frozen, take them out from the freezer and let them sit at room temperature for a few minutes to slightly soften, making them easier to blend.

3. In a blender, add the frozen banana slices, 1/4 cup of unsweetened almond milk, and one tablespoon of honey (if desired for added sweetness).

4. Optionally, add 1/2 teaspoon of vanilla extract for extra flavor.

5. Blend the mixture until it becomes smooth and creamy. You may need to stop and scrape down the sides of the blender a few times to ensure even blending.

6. Once the mixture is creamy and resembles ice cream, stop blending.

7. Scoop the Banana Ice Cream into bowls or serving dishes.

8. If desired, garnish with sliced almonds for added texture and flavor.

9. Serve the ice cream immediately. It has a soft-serve consistency right after blending.

Nutritional Information (Per Serving):

- Carbohydrates: 38g

- Fats: 1g

- Fiber: 4g

- Sodium: 1mg

- Protein: 1g

Chia Seed Pudding with Mango

Prep Time: 5 minutes
Cook Time: 0 minutes
Number of Servings: 4 servings

Ingredients:

- 1/2 cup chia seeds

- 2 cups unsweetened coconut milk

- 2 tablespoons honey (optional)

- 1 teaspoon vanilla extract

- 2 ripe mangoes, peeled, pitted, and diced

- Fresh mint leaves for garnish (optional)

Instructions:

1. In a mixing bowl, add 1/2 cup of chia seeds, two cups of unsweetened coconut milk, two tablespoons of honey (if desired for added sweetness), and one teaspoon of vanilla extract. Stir until well combined.

2. Allow the chia seed mixture to sit for about 5 minutes, then stir again to prevent clumping. Let it sit for another 10 minutes, stirring occasionally until it thickens to a pudding-like consistency.

3. While the chia seed pudding is thickening, peel, pit, and dice 2 ripe mangoes.

4. Once the chia seed pudding has thickened, divide it into four serving dishes or glasses.

5. Top each serving of chia seed pudding with the diced mango.

6. If desired, garnish with fresh mint leaves for a burst of color and flavor.

7. Serve the Chia Seed Pudding with Mango immediately, or refrigerate until ready to enjoy.

Nutritional Information (Per Serving):

- Carbohydrates: 40g
- Fats: 14g
- Fiber: 12g
- Sodium: 20mg
- Protein: 6g

Baked Pear with Caramel Drizzle

Prep Time: 10 minutes
Cook Time: 30 minutes
Number of Servings: 4 servings

Ingredients:

For the Baked Pears:

- 4 ripe pears
- 2 tablespoons honey
- 1 teaspoon ground cinnamon
- 1/4 cup chopped walnuts (optional)
- 1/4 cup gluten-free rolled oats
- 1 tablespoon unsalted butter (or dairy-free alternative)
- Pinch of salt

For the Caramel Drizzle:

- 1/4 cup honey
- 2 tablespoons unsalted butter (or dairy-free alternative)
- Pinch of salt

Instructions:

1. Turn on your oven and set it to 375°F (190°C).

2. Wash and peel 4 ripe pears. Cut them in half lengthwise and take out the cores. Place the pear halves in a baking dish, cut side up.

3. In a small bowl, add two tablespoons of honey and one teaspoon of ground cinnamon. Mix sufficiently to create a cinnamon-honey glaze.

4. Drizzle the cinnamon-honey glaze over the pear halves, ensuring each one is coated evenly.

5. In a separate bowl, add 1/4 cup of chopped walnuts (if using), 1/4 cup of gluten-free rolled oats, one tablespoon of unsalted butter (or dairy-free alternative), and a pinch of salt. Mix until the ingredients are well combined.

6. Spoon the walnut and oat mixture evenly onto each pear half.

7. Cover the baking dish with aluminum foil and bake in the preheated oven for 20 minutes.

8. After 20 minutes, take out the foil and bake for an extra 10 minutes or until the pears are tender and the topping is golden brown.

9. While the pears are baking, prepare the caramel drizzle. In a small saucepan, add 1/4 cup of honey, two tablespoons of unsalted butter (or dairy-free alternative), and a pinch of salt. Heat over low heat, stirring constantly, until the mixture is smooth and slightly thickened. Take it out from heat.

10. Once the pears are done baking, take them out from the oven and let them cool slightly.

11. Drizzle the caramel sauce over the baked pears.

12. Serve the Baked Pear with Caramel Drizzle warm, optionally with a scoop of vanilla ice cream or a dollop of yogurt for added richness.

Nutritional Information (Per Serving):

- Carbohydrates: 55g

- Fats: 14g

- Fiber: 7g

- Sodium: 96mg

- Protein: 2g

Almond Flour Blueberry Muffins

Prep Time: 15 minutes
Cook Time: 25 minutes
Number of Servings: 12 muffins

Ingredients:

- 2 cups almond flour

- 1/4 cup coconut flour

- 1/4 cup honey

- 1/4 cup melted coconut oil

- 3 large eggs

- 1/2 teaspoon baking soda

- 1/4 teaspoon salt

- 1 teaspoon vanilla extract

- 1 cup fresh blueberries

Instructions:

1. Turn on your oven and set it to 350°F (175°C). Line a muffin tin with paper liners or grease it with a bit of coconut oil to prevent sticking.

2. In a large mixing bowl, add two cups of almond flour and 1/4 cup of coconut flour.

3. In a separate bowl, whisk 1/4 cup of honey, 1/4 cup of melted coconut oil, 3 large eggs, 1/2 teaspoon of baking soda, 1/4 teaspoon of salt, and one teaspoon of vanilla extract.

4. Pour the wet ingredients into the dry ingredients and stir until well combined.

5. Gently fold in one cup of fresh blueberries into the muffin batter.

6. Using an ice cream scoop or spoon, divide the batter evenly among the 12 muffin cups in the tin.

7. Bake in the preheated oven for about 20-25 minutes or until a toothpick inserted into the center of a muffin comes out clean.

8. Once done, take out the muffins from the oven and allow them to cool in the tin for a few minutes before transferring them to a wire rack to cool completely.

9. Serve these Almond Flour Blueberry Muffins as a delightful and gastroparesis-friendly treat.

Nutritional Information (Per Serving - 1 Muffin):

- Carbohydrates: 13g

- Fats: 10g

- Fiber: 3g

- Sodium: 97mg

- Protein: 5g

Coconut Milk Rice Pudding

Prep Time: 5 minutes
Cook Time: 30 minutes
Number of Servings: 4 servings

Ingredients:

- 1 cup white rice

- 2 cups unsweetened coconut milk

- 1/4 cup honey (or to taste)

- 1/2 teaspoon vanilla extract

- Pinch of salt

- Ground cinnamon for garnish (optional)

- Shredded coconut for garnish (optional)

Instructions:

1. Rinse one cup of white rice under cold water until the water runs clear. Drain well.

2. In a medium-sized saucepan, add the rinsed rice, two cups of unsweetened coconut milk, 1/4 cup of honey, 1/2 teaspoon of vanilla extract, and a pinch of salt.

3. Place the saucepan over medium heat and bring the mixture to a gentle boil. Stir occasionally to prevent the rice from sticking to the bottom of the pan.

4. Once it starts boiling, reduce the heat to low and let the rice simmer for approximately 20-25 minutes, or until the rice is cooked and the mixture has thickened to a creamy consistency.

5. Take out the saucepan from the heat and let the rice pudding cool slightly.

6. Divide the Coconut Milk Rice Pudding into four serving bowls.

7. If desired, garnish with a sprinkle of ground cinnamon and shredded coconut for added flavor and texture.

8. Serve the rice pudding warm, optionally with additional honey for sweetness.

Nutritional Information (Per Serving):

- Carbohydrates: 59g

- Fats: 13g

- Fiber: 1g

- Sodium: 30mg

- Protein: 3g

Chocolate Avocado Mousse

Prep Time: 10 minutes
Cook Time: 0 minutes
Number of Servings: 4 servings

Ingredients:

- 2 ripe avocados, peeled and pitted

- 1/2 cup unsweetened cocoa powder
- 1/4 cup honey (or to taste)
- 1/4 cup unsweetened almond milk
- 1 teaspoon vanilla extract
- Pinch of salt
- Fresh berries for garnish (optional)

Instructions:

1. In a food processor or blender, add 2 ripe avocados, 1/2 cup of unsweetened cocoa powder, 1/4 cup of honey (adjust to taste), 1/4 cup of unsweetened almond milk, one teaspoon of vanilla extract, and a pinch of salt.

2. Blend the mixture until it becomes smooth and creamy. You may need to stop and scrape down the sides of the blender or processor a few times to ensure even blending.

3. Once the Chocolate Avocado Mousse is smooth and free of lumps, stop blending.

4. Divide the mousse into four individual serving cups or glasses.

5. If desired, garnish each serving with fresh berries for a burst of flavor and color.

6. Refrigerate the mousse for at least 30 minutes before serving to chill and firm up slightly.

7. Serve the Chocolate Avocado Mousse chilled as a rich and satisfying dessert.

Nutritional Information (Per Serving):

- Carbohydrates: 34g
- Fats: 15g
- Fiber: 9g
- Sodium: 26mg
- Protein: 5g

Pumpkin Pie with a Gluten-Free Crust

Prep Time: 15 minutes
Cook Time: 55 minutes
Number of Servings: 8 servings

Ingredients:

For the Gluten-Free Crust:

- 1 1/2 cups gluten-free all-purpose flour

- 1/2 cup cold unsalted butter (or dairy-free alternative), diced

- 1/4 cup ice-cold water

- 1/4 teaspoon salt

For the Pumpkin Filling:

- 1 15-ounce can pumpkin puree

- 1/2 cup coconut milk (full-fat)

- 1/2 cup honey (or to taste)

- 2 large eggs

- 1 teaspoon ground cinnamon

- 1/2 teaspoon ground nutmeg

- 1/4 teaspoon ground cloves

- 1/4 teaspoon salt

- 1 teaspoon vanilla extract

Instructions:

For the Gluten-Free Crust:

1. In a food processor, add 1 1/2 cups of gluten-free all-purpose flour and 1/4 teaspoon of salt.

2. Add 1/2 cup of cold, diced unsalted butter (or dairy-free alternative) to the food processor.

3. Pulse the mixture until it resembles coarse crumbs.

4. With the food processor running, slowly add 1/4 cup of ice-cold water until the dough comes together and forms a ball.

5. Turn the dough out onto a floured surface and shape it into a disk. Wrap it in plastic wrap and refrigerate for at least 30 minutes.

For the Pumpkin Filling:

6. Turn on your oven and set it to 375°F (190°C).

7. In a mixing bowl, add 1 15-ounce can of pumpkin puree, 1/2 cup of coconut milk, 1/2 cup of honey (adjust to taste), 2 large eggs, one teaspoon of ground cinnamon, 1/2 teaspoon of ground nutmeg, 1/4 teaspoon of ground cloves, 1/4 teaspoon of salt, and one teaspoon of vanilla extract. Mix until well combined.

Assembling the Pie:

8. Roll out the chilled gluten-free dough on a floured surface to fit a 9-inch (23 cm) pie dish.

9. Place the rolled-out dough into the pie dish and trim any excess. Crimp the edges with a fork or your fingers for a decorative finish.

10. Pour the prepared pumpkin filling into the pie crust.

11. Bake in the preheated oven for approximately 45-55 minutes or until the center is set and a toothpick inserted into the filling comes out clean.

12. Take out the pumpkin pie from the oven and allow it to cool completely before serving.

Nutritional Information (Per Serving):

- Carbohydrates: 44g
- Fats: 22g
- Fiber: 3g
- Sodium: 268mg
- Protein: 4g

BEVERAGES

Minty Cucumber and Melon Cooler

Prep Time: 15 minutes
Cook Time: 0 minutes
Number of Servings: 2

Ingredients:

- 1 cup diced cucumber
- 1 cup diced honeydew melon
- 1/4 cup fresh mint leaves
- 1/2 cup crushed ice
- 1/4 cup plain yogurt (ensure it's low-fat for gastroparesis)
- 1 tablespoon honey
- 1/2 teaspoon fresh ginger, grated
- A pinch of salt

Instructions:

1. Start by preparing your ingredients. Wash and peel the cucumber, then dice it into small pieces. Dice the honeydew melon as well, removing the seeds and rind.

2. In a blender, add the diced cucumber, diced honeydew melon, fresh mint leaves, crushed ice, low-fat plain yogurt, honey, grated fresh ginger, and a pinch of salt.

3. Blend everything until it becomes a smooth and creamy mixture, ensuring there are no lumps.

4. Taste the mixture and adjust the sweetness with more honey if desired. You can also add a touch more salt or ginger for extra flavor, based on your preferences and dietary needs.

5. Once your Minty Cucumber and Melon Cooler is perfectly blended and flavored, pour it into glasses.

6. Optionally, garnish with a sprig of fresh mint or a cucumber slice for an elegant presentation.

7. Serve immediately and enjoy your refreshing and gastroparesis-friendly cooler!

Nutritional Information (per serving):

- Carbs: 20 grams

- Fats: 1 gram

- Fiber: 2 grams

- Sodium: 80 milligrams

- Protein: 2 grams

Raspberry Lemonade

Prep Time: 10 minutes
Cook Time: 0 minutes
Number of Servings: 4

Ingredients:

- 1 cup fresh raspberries

- 1/2 cup freshly squeezed lemon juice (from about 4-5 lemons)

- 1/4 cup honey (adjust to taste or use a sugar substitute suitable for gastroparesis)

- 4 cups cold water

- Ice cubes

- Lemon slices and fresh raspberries for garnish

Instructions:

1. Begin by preparing your ingredients. Wash the fresh raspberries and set them aside.

2. Squeeze enough lemons to yield 1/2 cup of freshly squeezed lemon juice. This typically requires 4-5 lemons, depending on their size.

3. In a blender, add the fresh raspberries, freshly squeezed lemon juice, and honey (or a suitable gastroparesis-friendly sugar substitute).

4. Blend the mixture until the raspberries are fully pureed, and the mixture is smooth.

5. Strain the raspberry and lemon mixture through a fine-mesh sieve into a pitcher to remove any seeds or pulp.

6. Add 4 cups of cold water to the pitcher and stir sufficiently to combine.

7. Taste the raspberry lemonade and adjust the sweetness with more honey or sugar substitute if needed.

8. Fill glasses with ice cubes and pour the raspberry lemonade over the ice.

9. Garnish each glass with a lemon slice and a few fresh raspberries.

10. Serve immediately and enjoy your refreshing Raspberry Lemonade!

Nutritional Information (per serving):

- Carbs: 20 grams

- Fats: 0 grams

- Fiber: 2 grams

- Sodium: 10 milligrams

- Protein: 0 grams

Spinach and Pineapple Smoothie

Prep Time: 10 minutes
Cook Time: 0 minutes
Number of Servings: 2

Ingredients:

- 2 cups fresh spinach leaves

- 1 cup diced pineapple (canned in juice, drained)
- 1 medium ripe banana
- 1/2 cup low-fat plain yogurt (ensure it's suitable for gastroparesis)
- 1/2 cup cold water
- 1 tablespoon honey (adjust to taste or use a suitable gastroparesis-friendly sugar substitute)
- Ice cubes (optional)

Instructions:

1. Begin by preparing your ingredients. Wash the fresh spinach leaves thoroughly and set them aside.

2. Dice the pineapple into small pieces, ensuring it's drained if it was canned in juice.

3. Peel the ripe banana and break it into smaller chunks for easier blending.

4. In a blender, add the fresh spinach leaves, diced pineapple, banana chunks, low-fat plain yogurt (suitable for gastroparesis), and cold water.

5. Blend the mixture until it's smooth and all ingredients are well combined. If you prefer a colder smoothie, you can also add a few ice cubes at this stage.

6. Taste the smoothie and adjust the sweetness with honey or a gastroparesis-friendly sugar substitute according to your preferences.

7. Blend once more to incorporate the sweetness.

8. Pour the Spinach and Pineapple Smoothie into glasses and serve immediately.

Nutritional Information (per serving):

- Carbs: 30 grams
- Fats: 1 gram
- Fiber: 4 grams

- Sodium: 50 milligrams

- Protein: 4 grams

Blueberry and Lavender Infused Water

Prep Time: 5 minutes
Cook Time: 0 minutes
Number of Servings: 4

Ingredients:

- 2 cups fresh blueberries

- 2 tablespoons dried lavender buds

- 4 cups cold water

- Ice cubes (optional)

Instructions:

1. Begin by preparing your ingredients. Rinse the fresh blueberries thoroughly and set them aside.

2. In a small bowl, add the dried lavender buds with 1/2 cup of cold water. Allow them to steep for about 5 minutes to create a lavender-infused water.

3. In a pitcher, add the fresh blueberries.

4. Once the lavender-infused water has steeped, strain it to take out the lavender buds, then add the infused water to the pitcher with the blueberries.

5. Add the remaining 3 1/2 cups of cold water to the pitcher.

6. If you prefer a colder infusion, you can also add ice cubes to the pitcher at this stage.

7. Stir the mixture gently to combine the blueberries and lavender-infused water.

8. Allow the Blueberry and Lavender Infused Water to sit in the refrigerator for at least 30 minutes to let the flavors meld together.

9. When serving, you can add a few fresh blueberries and a sprig of fresh lavender for garnish if desired.

10. Serve the infused water in glasses with ice cubes, and enjoy its subtle fruity and floral flavors!

Nutritional Information (per serving):

- Carbs: 10 grams

- Fats: 0 grams

- Fiber: 2 grams

- Sodium: 5 milligrams

- Protein: 0 grams

Golden Milk Iced Latte

Prep Time: 5 minutes
Cook Time: 0 minutes
Number of Servings: 2

Ingredients:

- 2 cups unsweetened almond milk (ensure it's low-fat for gastroparesis)

- 2 teaspoons ground turmeric

- 1/2 teaspoon ground cinnamon

- 1/4 teaspoon ground ginger

- 1/4 teaspoon ground cardamom

- 1/8 teaspoon ground black pepper

- 1 tablespoon honey (adjust to taste or use a suitable gastroparesis-friendly sugar substitute)

- 2 cups ice cubes

Instructions:

1. Start by preparing your ingredients. Ensure you have two cups of unsweetened almond milk, and make sure it's low-fat to accommodate a gastroparesis diet.

2. In a small bowl, add the ground turmeric, ground cinnamon, ground ginger, ground cardamom, and ground black pepper. Mix them well to create your golden milk spice blend.

3. In a blender, add the almond milk and the spice blend you just prepared.

4. Blend the mixture until the spices are well incorporated into the almond milk.

5. Taste the mixture and adjust the sweetness with honey or a gastroparesis-friendly sugar substitute according to your preferences.

6. Add the ice cubes to the blender and blend again until the mixture becomes smooth and frothy.

7. Pour the Golden Milk Iced Latte into glasses and serve immediately.

8. Optionally, you can sprinkle a pinch of ground turmeric or cinnamon on top for garnish.

9. Enjoy your refreshing and gastroparesis-friendly Golden Milk Iced Latte!

Nutritional Information (per serving):

- Carbs: 8 grams

- Fats: 2 grams

- Fiber: 1 gram

- Sodium: 180 milligrams

- Protein: 1 gram

Cranberry and Orange Mocktail

Prep Time: 10 minutes
Cook Time: 0 minutes
Number of Servings: 2

Ingredients:

- 1 cup unsweetened cranberry juice

- 1/2 cup freshly squeezed orange juice (from about 2 oranges)
- 1/4 cup cold water
- 1 tablespoon honey (adjust to taste or use a suitable gastroparesis-friendly sugar substitute)
- Ice cubes
- Orange slices and fresh cranberries for garnish

Instructions:

1. Begin by preparing your ingredients. Squeeze enough oranges to yield 1/2 cup of freshly squeezed orange juice (approximately 2 oranges).

2. In a pitcher, add the unsweetened cranberry juice, freshly squeezed orange juice, and cold water.

3. Stir in the honey (or a gastroparesis-friendly sugar substitute) to sweeten the mocktail. Adjust the sweetness to your preference.

4. Fill glasses with ice cubes.

5. Pour the Cranberry and Orange Mocktail over the ice cubes in each glass.

6. Optionally, garnish each glass with a slice of orange and a few fresh cranberries for a festive touch.

7. Stir gently to combine the flavors.

8. Serve immediately and enjoy your gastroparesis-friendly Cranberry and Orange Mocktail!

Nutritional Information (per serving):

- Carbs: 25 grams
- Fats: 0 grams
- Fiber: 1 gram
- Sodium: 5 milligrams
- Protein: 0 grams

Fresh Ginger and Lemon Tea

Prep Time: 5 minutes
Cook Time: 10 minutes
Number of Servings: 2

Ingredients:

- 2 cups water

- 2 tablespoons fresh ginger, thinly sliced

- 2 tablespoons freshly squeezed lemon juice (from about 1 lemon)

- 1 tablespoon honey (adjust to taste or use a suitable gastroparesis-friendly sugar substitute)

- Lemon slices and fresh ginger slices for garnish

Instructions:

1. Begin by preparing your ingredients. Thinly slice two tablespoons of fresh ginger and set them aside.

2. In a saucepan, add two cups of water and the sliced fresh ginger.

3. Bring the water to a boil over medium-high heat.

4. Once the water is boiling, reduce the heat to low, cover the saucepan, and let the ginger simmer in the water for about 10 minutes. This will infuse the water with ginger flavor.

5. After 10 minutes, take out the saucepan from the heat and strain the ginger slices from the water. You should now have ginger-infused hot water.

6. Stir in the freshly squeezed lemon juice and honey (or a gastroparesis-friendly sugar substitute) into the ginger-infused hot water. Adjust the sweetness to your preference.

7. Pour the Fresh Ginger and Lemon Tea into cups.

8. Optionally, garnish each cup with a slice of lemon and a thin slice of fresh ginger for added flavor and presentation.

9. Allow the tea to cool slightly, then serve and enjoy your soothing and gastroparesis-friendly Fresh Ginger and Lemon Tea!

Nutritional Information (per serving):

- Carbs: 7 grams

- Fats: 0 grams

- Fiber: 0 grams

- Sodium: 5 milligrams

- Protein: 0 grams

Papaya and Mango Smoothie

Prep Time: 10 minutes
Cook Time: 0 minutes
Number of Servings: 2

Ingredients:

- 1 cup diced ripe papaya

- 1 cup diced ripe mango

- 1/2 cup low-fat plain yogurt (ensure it's suitable for gastroparesis)

- 1/2 cup cold water

- 1 tablespoon honey (adjust to taste or use a suitable gastroparesis-friendly sugar substitute)

- Ice cubes (optional)

Instructions:

1. Begin by preparing your ingredients. Peel, seed, and dice the ripe papaya, and do the same for the ripe mango.

2. In a blender, add the diced papaya, diced mango, low-fat plain yogurt (suitable for gastroparesis), and cold water.

3. Blend the mixture until it's smooth and all ingredients are well combined.

4. Taste the smoothie and adjust the sweetness with honey or a gastroparesis-friendly sugar substitute according to your preferences.

5. If you prefer a colder smoothie, you can also add ice cubes to the blender at this stage and blend until smooth.

6. Pour the Papaya and Mango Smoothie into glasses.

7. Serve immediately, and if desired, garnish with a small piece of papaya or mango for a decorative touch.

8. Enjoy your refreshing and gastroparesis-friendly Papaya and Mango Smoothie!

Nutritional Information (per serving):

- Carbs: 30 grams

- Fats: 1 gram

- Fiber: 3 grams

- Sodium: 50 milligrams

- Protein: 3 grams

Sparkling Lavender Lemonade

Prep Time: 15 minutes
Cook Time: 0 minutes
Number of Servings: 4

Ingredients:

- 2 cups water

- 2 tablespoons dried lavender buds

- 1 cup freshly squeezed lemon juice (from about 4-5 lemons)

- 1/2 cup honey (adjust to taste or use a suitable gastroparesis-friendly sugar substitute)

- 2 cups sparkling water (unsweetened)

- Ice cubes

- Lemon slices and fresh lavender sprigs for garnish

Instructions:

1. Begin by preparing your ingredients. Squeeze enough lemons to yield one cup of freshly squeezed lemon juice (approximately 4-5 lemons).

2. In a small saucepan, add two cups of water and the dried lavender buds.

3. Bring the water to a gentle boil over medium heat, then reduce the heat to low, cover, and let it simmer for about 5 minutes. This will create a lavender-infused water.

4. After 5 minutes, take out the saucepan from the heat and strain out the lavender buds, leaving you with lavender-infused hot water.

5. In a pitcher, add the freshly squeezed lemon juice and honey (or a gastroparesis-friendly sugar substitute). Stir sufficiently to dissolve the honey.

6. Pour the lavender-infused hot water into the pitcher with the lemon juice and honey mixture. Stir to combine.

7. Fill the pitcher with ice cubes to cool the mixture down.

8. Once the mixture has cooled, slowly pour in the sparkling water. Be gentle to preserve the carbonation.

9. Taste the Sparkling Lavender Lemonade and adjust the sweetness with more honey or sugar substitute if desired.

10. Serve the lemonade in glasses filled with ice cubes.

11. Optionally, garnish each glass with a slice of lemon and a sprig of fresh lavender for an elegant presentation.

12. Enjoy your sparkling and gastroparesis-friendly Lavender Lemonade!

Nutritional Information (per serving):

- Carbs: 30 grams

- Fats: 0 grams

- Fiber: 1 gram

- Sodium: 20 milligrams

- Protein: 0 grams

Green Tea Latte with Almond Milk

Prep Time: 5 minutes
Cook Time: 5 minutes
Number of Servings: 2

Ingredients:

- 2 cups unsweetened almond milk (ensure it's low-fat for gastroparesis)

- 2 green tea bags

- 2 tablespoons honey (adjust to taste or use a suitable gastroparesis-friendly sugar substitute)

- 1/4 teaspoon pure vanilla extract

- Ground cinnamon for garnish (optional)

Instructions:

1. Begin by preparing your ingredients. Ensure you have two cups of unsweetened almond milk, and make sure it's low-fat to accommodate a gastroparesis diet.

2. In a small saucepan, heat the almond milk over medium-low heat until it's steaming but not boiling. Be careful not to scorch the milk.

3. While the almond milk is heating, place the green tea bags in the saucepan with the almond milk. Let them steep for 3-5 minutes, depending on your desired tea strength.

4. Take out the saucepan from the heat and carefully take out the green tea bags.

5. Stir in the honey (or a gastroparesis-friendly sugar substitute) and pure vanilla extract into the green tea-infused almond milk. Adjust the sweetness to your preference.

6. Pour the Green Tea Latte with Almond Milk into cups.

7. Optionally, sprinkle a pinch of ground cinnamon on top for garnish, if desired.

8. Serve immediately and enjoy your soothing and gastroparesis-friendly Green Tea Latte with Almond Milk!

Nutritional Information (per serving):

- Carbs: 20 grams

- Fats: 2 grams

- Fiber: 1 gram

- Sodium: 180 milligrams

- Protein: 1 gram

Lemon Water with Fresh Mint

Prep Time: 5 minutes
Cook Time: 0 minutes
Number of Servings: 2

Ingredients:

- 2 cups cold water

- 1 lemon, sliced

- 8-10 fresh mint leaves

- 1 tablespoon honey (adjust to taste or use a suitable gastroparesis-friendly sugar substitute)

- Ice cubes (optional)

Instructions:

1. Begin by preparing your ingredients. Wash the lemon thoroughly and slice it.

2. In a pitcher, add the cold water and lemon slices.

3. Gently bruise the fresh mint leaves by lightly pressing them between your fingers to release their flavor, and then add them to the pitcher with the lemon and water.

4. Stir in the honey (or a gastroparesis-friendly sugar substitute) to sweeten the lemon water. Adjust the sweetness to your preference.

5. If you prefer a colder drink, you can add ice cubes to the pitcher.

6. Stir the mixture well to ensure the honey is fully dissolved.

7. Allow the Lemon Water with Fresh Mint to sit for a few minutes to let the flavors meld together.

8. Serve the lemon water in glasses, ensuring that each glass has lemon slices and fresh mint leaves.

9. Enjoy your refreshing and gastroparesis-friendly Lemon Water with Fresh Mint!

Nutritional Information (per serving):

- Carbs: 15 grams

- Fats: 0 grams

- Fiber: 2 grams

- Sodium: 5 milligrams

- Protein: 0 grams

Cucumber and Mint Infused Water

Prep Time: 5 minutes
Cook Time: 0 minutes
Number of Servings: 2

Ingredients:

- 2 cups cold water

- 1/2 cucumber, thinly sliced

- 10-12 fresh mint leaves

- Ice cubes (optional)

Instructions:

1. Begin by preparing your ingredients. Wash the cucumber thoroughly and slice it thinly.

2. In a pitcher, add the cold water, thinly sliced cucumber, and fresh mint leaves.

3. If you prefer a colder infused water, you can add ice cubes to the pitcher.

4. Stir the mixture gently to distribute the cucumber and mint flavors throughout the water.

5. Allow the Cucumber and Mint Infused Water to sit for a few minutes to allow the flavors to meld together.

6. Serve the infused water in glasses, ensuring that each glass has cucumber slices and fresh mint leaves for a visually appealing and flavorful experience.

7. Enjoy your refreshing and gastroparesis-friendly Cucumber and Mint Infused Water!

Nutritional Information (per serving):

- Carbs: 3 grams

- Fats: 0 grams

- Fiber: 1 gram

- Sodium: 10 milligrams

- Protein: 0 grams

Berry Smoothie with Spinach
Prep Time: 5 minutes
Cook Time: 0 minutes
Number of Servings: 2

Ingredients:

- 1 cup fresh or frozen mixed berries (such as strawberries, blueberries, and raspberries)

- 1 cup fresh spinach leaves

- 1/2 cup low-fat plain yogurt (ensure it's suitable for gastroparesis)

- 1/2 cup cold water

- 1 tablespoon honey (adjust to taste or use a suitable gastroparesis-friendly sugar substitute)

- Ice cubes (optional)

Instructions:

1. Begin by preparing your ingredients. Wash the fresh spinach leaves thoroughly and set them aside.

2. In a blender, add the fresh or frozen mixed berries, fresh spinach leaves, low-fat plain yogurt (suitable for gastroparesis), and cold water.

3. Blend the mixture until it's smooth and all ingredients are well combined.

4. Taste the smoothie and adjust the sweetness with honey or a gastroparesis-friendly sugar substitute according to your preferences.

5. If you prefer a colder smoothie, you can also add ice cubes to the blender at this stage and blend until smooth.

6. Pour the Berry Smoothie with Spinach into glasses.

7. Serve immediately and enjoy your nutrient-packed and gastroparesis-friendly Berry Smoothie with Spinach!

Nutritional Information (per serving):

- Carbs: 20 grams

- Fats: 1 gram

- Fiber: 4 grams

- Sodium: 60 milligrams

- Protein: 3 grams

Iced Green Tea with Honey

Prep Time: 5 minutes
Cook Time: 5 minutes (plus cooling time)
Number of Servings: 2

Ingredients:

- 2 green tea bags

- 2 cups boiling water

- 2 tablespoons honey (adjust to taste or use a suitable gastroparesis-friendly sugar substitute)

- Ice cubes

- Lemon slices for garnish (optional)

Instructions:

1. Begin by preparing your ingredients. Place 2 green tea bags in a heatproof pitcher or jug.

2. Pour two cups of boiling water over the tea bags.

3. Allow the tea bags to steep in the hot water for about 5 minutes or until you reach your desired tea strength. You can adjust the steeping time to your preference.

4. Once the tea has steeped, take out the tea bags and discard them.

5. Stir in the honey (or a gastroparesis-friendly sugar substitute) into the hot tea until it's fully dissolved.

6. Let the sweetened tea cool to room temperature, and then refrigerate it until it's cold. This will take approximately 1-2 hours.

7. When ready to serve, fill glasses with ice cubes.

8. Pour the chilled Iced Green Tea with Honey over the ice cubes in each glass.

9. Optionally, garnish each glass with a slice of lemon for added flavor and presentation.

10. Serve immediately and enjoy your refreshing and gastroparesis-friendly Iced Green Tea with Honey!

Nutritional Information (per serving):

- Carbs: 20 grams
- Fats: 0 grams
- Fiber: 0 grams
- Sodium: 10 milligrams
- Protein: 0 grams

Golden Milk (Turmeric Latte)

Prep Time: 5 minutes
Cook Time: 10 minutes
Number of Servings: 2

Ingredients:

- 2 cups unsweetened almond milk (ensure it's low-fat for gastroparesis)
- 1 teaspoon ground turmeric
- 1/2 teaspoon ground cinnamon
- 1/4 teaspoon ground ginger
- 1/4 teaspoon ground cardamom
- 1/8 teaspoon ground black pepper
- 1 tablespoon honey (adjust to taste or use a suitable gastroparesis-friendly sugar substitute)
- 1/2 teaspoon pure vanilla extract

Instructions:

1. Begin by preparing your ingredients. Ensure you have two cups of unsweetened almond milk, and make sure it's low-fat to accommodate a gastroparesis diet.

2. In a small saucepan, add the almond milk over medium-low heat. Warm the almond milk, but do not bring it to a boil. Keep an eye on it to prevent scorching.

3. While the almond milk is warming, in a separate bowl, add the ground turmeric, ground cinnamon, ground ginger, ground cardamom, and ground black pepper to create your golden milk spice blend.

4. Once the almond milk is warm, whisk in the golden milk spice blend, ensuring it's fully dissolved.

5. Stir in the honey (or a gastroparesis-friendly sugar substitute) and pure vanilla extract. Adjust the sweetness to your preference.

6. Continue to heat the mixture over low heat for about 5-7 minutes, stirring occasionally. This allows the flavors to meld together.

7. Take out the saucepan from heat when the Golden Milk is hot, but not boiling.

8. Pour the Golden Milk (Turmeric Latte) into mugs.

9. Serve immediately and enjoy the soothing and gastroparesis-friendly Golden Milk!

Nutritional Information (per serving):

- Carbs: 15 grams
- Fats: 2 grams
- Fiber: 0 grams
- Sodium: 180 milligrams
- Protein: 1 gram

Fresh Orange and Carrot Juice

Prep Time: 10 minutes
Cook Time: 0 minutes
Number of Servings: 2

Ingredients:

- 4 large carrots, washed and peeled
- 4 medium-sized oranges, peeled and segmented

- Ice cubes (optional)

Instructions:

1. Begin by preparing your ingredients. Wash and peel 4 large carrots.

2. Peel and segment 4 medium-sized oranges. Make sure to remove any seeds.

3. In a juicer or blender, add the peeled and segmented oranges.

4. Follow with the peeled carrots.

5. If you prefer a colder juice, you can add ice cubes to the blender at this stage.

6. Blend the mixture until it's smooth and all ingredients are well combined.

7. Optionally, you can strain the juice through a fine-mesh sieve to remove any remaining pulp, although leaving some pulp is suitable for a gastroparesis diet.

8. Pour the Fresh Orange and Carrot Juice into glasses.

9. Serve immediately and enjoy your refreshing and gastroparesis-friendly Fresh Orange and Carrot Juice!

Nutritional Information (per serving):

- Carbs: 30 grams

- Fats: 1 gram

- Fiber: 6 grams

- Sodium: 75 milligrams

- Protein: 2 grams

Cranberry and Raspberry Sparkling Water

Prep Time: 5 minutes
Cook Time: 0 minutes
Number of Servings: 2

Ingredients:

- 1 cup unsweetened cranberry juice
- 1/2 cup fresh raspberries
- 2 cups sparkling water (unsweetened)
- Ice cubes
- Fresh mint leaves for garnish (optional)

Instructions:

1. Begin by preparing your ingredients. Ensure you have one cup of unsweetened cranberry juice.

2. Wash and rinse 1/2 cup of fresh raspberries.

3. In a pitcher, add the unsweetened cranberry juice and the fresh raspberries.

4. Using a muddler or the back of a spoon, gently mash the raspberries to release their flavor into the cranberry juice.

5. Add ice cubes to the pitcher if you prefer a colder drink.

6. Slowly pour in two cups of sparkling water into the pitcher with the cranberry juice and mashed raspberries. Be gentle to preserve the carbonation.

7. Stir the mixture gently to combine the flavors.

8. Optionally, garnish each glass with a fresh mint leaf for added aroma and presentation.

9. Serve immediately, and enjoy your refreshing and gastroparesis-friendly Cranberry and Raspberry Sparkling Water!

Nutritional Information (per serving):

- Carbs: 20 grams
- Fats: 0 grams
- Fiber: 3 grams
- Sodium: 20 milligrams
- Protein: 1 gram

Chapter 12

30-Day Meal Plan

Here is a complete meal plan for 30 days, including breakfast, lunch, and dinner. You can adjust the portion sizes and ingredients to suit your diet and calorie needs.

Week 1

Day 1:

- Breakfast: Pumpkin Spice Smoothie
- Lunch: Creamy Spinach and Potato Soup
- Dinner: Lemon Dill Baked Cod

Day 2:

- Breakfast: Baked Quinoa Breakfast Bars
- Lunch: Shredded Carrot and Apple Salad
- Dinner: Turkey and Quinoa Stuffed Bell Peppers

Day 3:

- Breakfast: Coconut Rice Pudding
- Lunch: Tofu and Broccoli Slaw Salad
- Dinner: Creamy Chicken and Rice Casserole

Day 4:

- Breakfast: Scrambled Eggs with Fresh Dill
- Lunch: Pear and Walnut Salad
- Dinner: Zucchini and Carrot Noodles with Pesto

Day 5:

- Breakfast: Chia Seed and Raspberry Parfait
- Lunch: Roasted Red Pepper and Tomato Bisque
- Dinner: Ginger Teriyaki Tofu

Day 6:

- Breakfast: Creamy Polenta with Berries

- Lunch: Grape and Cottage Cheese Salad

- Dinner: Baked Eggplant Parmesan (Gluten-Free)

Day 7:

- Breakfast: Poached Chicken and Rice Soup

- Lunch: Caprese Salad with Balsamic Glaze

- Dinner: Spinach and Feta Stuffed Chicken Breast

Week 2
Day 8:

- Breakfast: Scrambled Eggs with Fresh Dill

- Lunch: Jicama and Cucumber Salad

- Dinner: Lentil and Butternut Squash Curry

Day 9:

- Breakfast: Creamy Peanut Butter Porridge

- Lunch: Thai-Inspired Cabbage Salad

- Dinner: Baked Trout with Herbed Butter

Day 10:

- Breakfast: Cinnamon Raisin French Toast (Gluten-Free)

- Lunch: Mixed Greens with Raspberry Walnut Vinaigrette

- Dinner: Shrimp Scampi with Zoodles

Day 11:

- Breakfast: Creamy Oatmeal with Mashed Banana

- Lunch: Mixed Greens with Grilled Chicken and Raspberry Vinaigrette

- Dinner: Baked Salmon with Lemon-Dill Sauce

Day 12:

- Breakfast: Scrambled Tofu with Spinach

- Lunch: Avocado and Grapefruit Salad
- Dinner: Turkey and Rice Casserole

Day 13:

- Breakfast: Baked Apples with Cinnamon
- Lunch: Quinoa and Roasted Vegetable Salad
- Dinner: Zucchini Noodles with Pesto

Day 14:

- Breakfast: Quinoa Porridge with Almond Butter
- Lunch: Cucumber and Mint Salad
- Dinner: Baked Cod with Herbed Butter

Week 3

Day 15:

- Breakfast: Ginger Carrot Smoothie
- Lunch: Tuna Salad with Greek Yogurt Dressing
- Dinner: Quiche with a Gluten-Free Crust

Day 16:

- Breakfast: Poached Egg with Steamed Asparagus
- Lunch: Beet and Orange Salad
- Dinner: Lemon Dill Baked Cod

Day 17:

- Breakfast: Blueberry Chia Pudding
- Lunch: Spinach and Strawberry Salad
- Dinner: Turkey and Quinoa Stuffed Bell Peppers

Day 18:

- Breakfast: Sweet Potato Hash Browns
- Lunch: Watermelon and Feta Salad
- Dinner: Creamy Chicken and Rice Casserole

Day 19:

- Breakfast: Pumpkin Spice Smoothie
- Lunch: Cilantro Lime Chicken Soup
- Dinner: Zucchini and Carrot Noodles with Pesto

Day 20:

- Breakfast: Baked Quinoa Breakfast Bars
- Lunch: Roasted Red Pepper and Tomato Bisque
- Dinner: Ginger Teriyaki Tofu

Day 21:

- Breakfast: Coconut Rice Pudding
- Lunch: Shrimp and Quinoa Chowder
- Dinner: Baked Eggplant Parmesan (Gluten-Free)

Week 4

Day 22:

- Breakfast: Scrambled Eggs with Fresh Dill
- Lunch: Creamy Parsnip and Apple Soup
- Dinner: Spinach and Feta Stuffed Chicken Breast

Day 23:

- Breakfast: Chia Seed and Raspberry Parfait
- Lunch: White Bean and Kale Soup
- Dinner: Lentil and Butternut Squash Curry

Day 24:

- Breakfast: Creamy Polenta with Berries
- Lunch: Creamy Mushroom and Rice Soup
- Dinner: Baked Trout with Herbed Butter

Day 25:

- Breakfast: Poached Chicken and Rice Soup

- Lunch: Sweet Potato and Leek Soup
- Dinner: Shrimp Scampi with Zoodles

Day 26:

- Breakfast: Spinach and Feta Omelette
- Lunch: Turkey Meatball Soup with Rice
- Dinner: Baked Salmon with Lemon-Dill Sauce

Day 27:

- Breakfast: Creamy Peanut Butter Porridge
- Lunch: Butternut Squash Soup with Ginger
- Dinner: Turkey and Rice Casserole

Day 28:

- Breakfast: Cinnamon Raisin French Toast (Gluten-Free)
- Lunch: Chicken and Rice Congee
- Dinner: Quiche with a Gluten-Free Crust

Day 29:

- Breakfast: Creamy Oatmeal with Mashed Banana
- Lunch: Creamy Tomato Soup with Rice
- Dinner: Zucchini Noodles with Pesto

Day 30:

- Breakfast: Scrambled Tofu with Spinach
- Lunch: Miso Soup with Silken Tofu
- Dinner: Lemon Dill Baked Cod

Conclusion

As we conclude our journey through *"The Complete Gastroparesis Cookbook,"* we hope you've found inspiration, knowledge, and a sense of control over your dietary choices and overall well-being. This cookbook showcases not only a variety of recipes but also the resilience, adaptability, and unwavering spirit of individuals who confront the challenges of gastroparesis on a daily basis.

Earlier in this cookbook, we explored the complexities of gastroparesis, including its causes, symptoms, diagnosis, and significant impact on eating habits. We have discussed the critical role of diet in managing this condition, focusing on symptom control, ease of digestion, blood sugar management, and prevention of malnutrition.

The motivation behind creating this cookbook was to offer individuals with gastroparesis and their caregivers a valuable resource. It's a resource that helps you make informed food choices and enjoy delicious, nourishing meals without worsening your condition.

We have discussed the significance of education, the importance of collaborating with healthcare professionals, and the benefits of maintaining a food diary. We have advised you to begin at a slow pace, try out different recipes, manage your portion sizes, and, above all, pay attention to your body.

Your journey towards better digestive health and improved quality of life is not a one-time event; it is a continuous process. We hope that the recipes and insights within these pages serve as a starting point for you to develop a satisfying and sustainable diet that is suitable for gastroparesis.

Remember that you are not alone in this journey. There is a community of individuals who can relate to the challenges you face, and the support and knowledge you gain from them are precious. By cultivating resilience, practicing patience, and utilizing the appropriate tools, it is possible to manage gastroparesis effectively. This will allow you to fully enjoy the experience of nourishing your body and savoring the sensory pleasures of each meal.

We hope you find a path to wellness that includes nourishing yourself, taking care of yourself, and enjoying delicious meals that meet your specific needs. Your health is important, and we are grateful to have been involved in your journey towards improving your life with gastroparesis.

Recipe Index

A

Almond Flour Banana Muffins 141

Almond Flour Blueberry Muffins 175

Almond Flour Chocolate Chip Cookies 156

Avocado and Grapefruit Salad 77

B

Baked Apple Chips 151

Baked Apples with Cinnamon 24

Baked Cinnamon Apple Slices 136

Baked Cinnamon Pears 158

Baked Cod with Herbed Butter 109

Baked Eggplant Parmesan (Gluten-Free) 97

Baked Pear with Caramel Drizzle 173

Baked Quinoa Breakfast Bars 10

Baked Salmon with Lemon-Dill Sauce 105

Baked Sweet Potato Fries 143

Baked Trout with Herbed Butter 102

Banana and Coconut Ice Cream 168

Banana and Peanut Butter Smoothie 147

Banana Ice Cream 170

Beet and Orange Salad 84

Berry Smoothie with Spinach 196

Blueberry and Lavender Infused Water 185

Blueberry Chia Pudding 30

Blueberry Crumble (Gluten-Free) 166

Boiled Edamame with Sea Salt 154

Butternut Squash Soup with Ginger 48

C

Caprese Salad with Balsamic Glaze 70

Carrot and Celery Sticks with Hummus 153

Cheddar Cheese Slices with Sliced Pear 144

Chia Seed and Coconut Pudding 157

Chia Seed and Raspberry Parfait 14

Chia Seed Pudding with Mango 172

Chicken and Rice Congee 50

Chocolate Avocado Brownies (Gluten-Free) 160

Chocolate Avocado Mousse 177

Cilantro Lime Chicken Soup 35

Cinnamon Raisin French Toast (Gluten-Free) 21

Coconut Milk Rice Pudding 176

Coconut Rice Pudding 12

Coconut Rice Pudding with Mango 161

Cottage Cheese with Pineapple 149

Cranberry and Orange Mocktail 187

Cranberry and Raspberry Sparkling Water 201

Creamy Cauliflower Soup 58

Creamy Chicken and Rice Casserole 92

Creamy Corn Pudding 123

Creamy Mushroom and Rice Soup 44

Creamy Oatmeal with Mashed Banana 22

Creamy Parsnip and Apple Soup 39

Creamy Peanut Butter Porridge 19

Creamy Polenta with Berries 15

Creamy Spinach and Potato Soup 34

Creamy Tomato Soup with Rice 52

Cucumber and Bell Pepper Sticks with Hummus 142

Cucumber and Mint Infused Water 195

Cucumber and Mint Salad 80

F

Fresh Ginger and Lemon Tea 189

Fresh Orange and Carrot Juice 200

G

Garlic Mashed Potatoes 124

Ginger Carrot Smoothie 27

Ginger Glazed Carrots 131

Ginger Teriyaki Tofu 95

Golden Milk (Turmeric Latte) 199

Golden Milk Iced Latte 186

Grape and Cottage Cheese Salad 68

Greek Yogurt Parfait with Kiwi 140

Greek Yogurt with Honey and Berries 150

Green Tea Latte with Almond Milk 193

Grilled Asparagus with Garlic Butter 119

I

Iced Green Tea with Honey 198

J

Jicama and Cucumber Salad 71

L

Lemon Chicken and Rice Soup 41

Lemon Dill Baked Cod 89

Lemon Herb Quinoa 132

Lemon Herb Quinoa Salad 116

Lemon Herb Quinoa Salad 118

Lemon Sorbet 163

Lemon Water with Fresh Mint 194

Lentil and Butternut Squash Curry 100

Lentil and Spinach Stew 56

M

Mashed Cauliflower with Chives 130

Mashed Sweet Potatoes with Cinnamon 113

Mashed Turnips with Chives 122

Minty Cucumber and Melon Cooler 181

Miso Soup with Silken Tofu 53

Mixed Greens with Grilled Chicken and Raspberry Vinaigrette 75

Mixed Greens with Raspberry Walnut Vinaigrette 74

P

Papaya and Mango Smoothie 190

Peach and Banana Smoothie 139

Pear and Walnut Salad 65

Poached Chicken and Rice Soup 17

Poached Egg with Steamed Asparagus 28

Potato Leek Soup with a Hint of Nutmeg 54

Pumpkin Pie with a Gluten-Free Crust 179

Pumpkin Spice Smoothie 9

Q

Quiche with a Gluten-Free Crust 110

Quinoa and Roasted Vegetable Salad 79

Quinoa Porridge with Almond Butter 26

R

Raspberry and Dark Chocolate Yogurt Cups 165

Raspberry Lemonade 182

Rice Cakes with Almond Butter 146

Rice Cakes with Cottage Cheese and Berries 137

Rice Pudding with Cinnamon 169

Roasted Beet and Arugula Salad 67

Roasted Brussels Sprouts with Pecans 114

Roasted Carrots with Dill 128

Roasted Chickpeas with Paprika 148

Roasted Pumpkin Seeds with Sea Salt 138

Roasted Red Pepper and Tomato Bisque 36

S

Sautéed Green Beans with Almonds 115

Sautéed Spinach with Garlic 127

Scrambled Eggs with Fresh Dill 13

Scrambled Tofu with Spinach 23

Shredded Carrot and Apple Salad 62

Shrimp and Quinoa Chowder 38

Shrimp Scampi with Zoodles 103

Sliced Cucumber with Yogurt Dill Sauce 134

Sparkling Lavender Lemonade 191

Spinach and Feta Omelette 18

Spinach and Feta Stuffed Chicken Breast 98

Spinach and Pineapple Smoothie 183

Spinach and Quinoa Salad with Lemon Dressing 61

Spinach and Strawberry Salad 85

Steamed Artichokes with Lemon Aioli 120

Steamed Broccoli with Almonds 126

Sweet Potato and Leek Soup 45

Sweet Potato Hash Browns 31

T

Thai-Inspired Cabbage Salad 72

Tofu and Broccoli Slaw Salad 64

Tuna Salad with Greek Yogurt Dressing 82

Turkey and Quinoa Stuffed Bell Peppers 90

Turkey and Rice Casserole 106

Turkey and Vegetable Broth 57

Turkey Meatball Soup with Rice 46

V

Vanilla Almond Milkshake 164

W

Watermelon and Feta Salad 87

Watermelon and Mint Skewers 145

White Bean and Kale Soup 42

Z

Zucchini and Carrot Noodles with Pesto 94

Zucchini Noodles with Pesto 108